How to get into
Graduate Entry Medical School

Dawn Sellars
Yolande Knight

How to get into Graduate Entry Medical School

Published in 2005 by Spine Publishing, part of Dr Prep Ltd, 35 Hills Road, Cambridge, CB2 1NT

British Library Cataloguing in Publication Data
A catalogue record for this book is available from the British Library.

ISBN 0-9551325-0-9

Cover design by Bruce Wilson

Contents

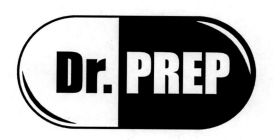

Contributors

Caroline Burchell BSc, MBBS
PRHO, Kingston Hospital

Yolande Knight BMedSc, PhD
Final year medical student, St George's, University of London
Honorary Fellow, Institute of Neurology

Eira Makepeace JP, BA (Rand), MA (Education)
Magistrate
Education Consultant
Director on the UCAS Board of Directors (1995 - 2003)

Phyllida Roe BA (Hons), BSc (Hons)
Head of Careers, The Princess Helena College (1987 - 1996)
First Year Medical Student, Peninsula University

Dawn Sellars MA (Cantab)
Final year medical student, St George's, University of London
Managing Director, Dr Prep Ltd

Bruce Wilson BSc, SRPara
Penultimate year medical student, St George's, University of London
Paramedic, London Ambulance Service

Acknowledgements

David Brewis MChem (Oxon)
Schoolmaster, St Paul's School
Company Director, QuizQuizQuiz Ltd

Simon Meller MB BS, DCH, FRCP, FRCPCH, LLB (Hons)
Postgraduate Student in Medical Ethics and Law
Formerly Consultant Paediatrician and Paediatric Oncologist

Adam Waldman BSc (Hons), MA, PhD, MBBChir, MRCP, FRCR
Consultant Neuroradiologist, Charing Cross Hospital
Honorary Senior Lecturer, Institute of Neurology, University College
London and Imperial College of Science Technology and Medicine

In compiling a book of this nature we have had to pool information from myriad sources. Numerous people have helped us in immeasurable ways. We would like to thank the above people, in addition to

Prof Peter Goadsby, Dr Miles Levy, Dr Jane Durkin, Dr Bishwajit Naha, Dr Pieter Van der Zee, Dr Gemma Way, Drs Richard and Rosie Wynne, Captain Stephen Penfold, William Ryder, James Wynne, Davina Hensman, Kate Diamond, Lindsey Ward, James d'Arcy, Karen Eccleshall, Caroline Weaver, Shirley Lyle, Elizabeth Ball, Farid Ahmed, the Foulkes Foundation and our family and friends.

FOREWORD

September 2005

Why do you want to be a doctor?
Earnest applicants always worry about the 'right' answer to this old chestnut before their interview at medical school. What are they looking for? How can I find out? If the internet has no answer, perhaps I should go to a bookstore or a library. This valuable little book goes a long way to providing some clues.

It was formative experiences in early childhood that directed me toward Medicine as a way of life. My GP was the nicest adult I had ever met, he had miraculous powers and my mother always gave him a cup of tea if he made a house call. At the age of seven, I contracted scarlet fever; at the time the treatment consisted of a month's rest in complete isolation in a fever hospital and, when I was finally released all *formites* - that is personal belongings that I had touched - had to be incinerated. The reason could never be explained to me, but I now understand that this was because there was no evidence base. 'Because the doctor says so' never cut much ice as far as I was concerned, but I was impudently ahead of my time. A desire to question the *status quo* is a good starting point, but the student needs to understand that 'it is not what you do, but the way that you do it'. A medical school applicant has even less licence to be impudent than the expert patient - even one who is seven years old!

Hospital consultants were aloof and mysterious pin-striped gentlemen that my GP regarded with awe. Much later, when I was a medical student, one such Consultant invited 'the firm' to a party at his mansion on Epsom Downs and to inspect his stud; it was only after we toured the stables that it was pointed out to me that we had seen the stud - I was expecting some kind of floor show after dinner. It was on this basis that I decided to become a Consultant, but in due course I discovered that this decision had been based on dodgy information and it never quite worked out the way I had imagined it would. Nonetheless, I have no regrets and I am still to be found encouraging young people to enter medicine if they have the aptitude and the determination.

The authors of this book clearly feel the same way as I do and, although they do not pretend that it is an easy option, they provide sound information on how to do it and a guide to help you through the maze. It is never too late to enter Medicine, but rather like having a baby, there are more difficult hurdles for mature graduate students than for school leavers; so if you are going to do it and for whatever reason, the sooner you get started the better. Unlike childbirth, in these days of equal opportunities it is equally possible, but equally difficult, for both sexes to succeed in Medicine - but beware, some medical schools are more equal than others. This book will help, but in the end it is the determined <u>and</u> informed individual who beats the system and gets in.

Simon Meller MB BS, DCH, FRCP, FRCPCH, LLB (Hons)
Postgraduate Student in Medical Ethics and Law
Formerly Consultant Paediatrician and Paediatric Oncologist

Introduction

Medicine is a rewarding profession offering a wide choice of careers. Many readers of this book will have had a burning desire to become a doctor for many years, whilst others will have developed the desire later on in life. Although in the past, 10-15% of those accepted onto standard entry MBBS courses in the UK have been graduates, many have previously felt unable to pursue their dream of medicine. The new, specifically designed graduate entry courses allow people to make this career decision in their 20s and 30s, when their motivation is less likely to be influenced by others, and when they have often gained vast life experience and transferable skills. Although a career that involves further specialist training for many years after graduation can be daunting for someone already that much older, the benefits of a vocation that combines mental stimulation with social interaction has an appeal that, for many, is unsurpassed.

Graduates from many different backgrounds are eligible to apply for a range of graduate entry medical courses. The diversity of their abilities and ages has understandably created many new approaches to selection. Entrance exams, supplementary application forms and novel interview structures often form part of graduate entry selection. Unfortunately, despite the trend towards widening access to medicine, the playing field is far from level, with some potentially good doctors falling at the first hurdles.

We are final year medical students on a graduate entry course and were successful in a number of entrance exams and interviews four years ago.

At that time we found it difficult, due to somewhat inaccessible and inadequate information, to know how to prepare for the entrance examinations and for graduate entry to medicine in general. We were fortunate in both having backgrounds heavily allied to medicine, in addition to some genuinely inspiring colleagues and friends. We recognised that many equally capable candidates did not have our fortunate, if not privileged, background. Therefore, we hope to pass on to you the wisdom of those same inspirational colleagues, as well as the knowledge and experience that we have gained through consultation with hundreds of graduate entry applicants to all fourteen graduate entry medical schools.

When we applied to graduate entry medicine there was no single source of comprehensive information like that provided in this book. Therefore, we have aimed to cover the breadth and depth of topics we would have wanted information on at that time. We have tried to structure the content of the book such that the reader can dip in and out of relevant topics where necessary, or peruse it from cover to cover if desired.

Contributions have been made by some insightful and generous colleagues, to whom we are most grateful.

This book is written for all graduate entry applicants, whether currently undergraduates, or older applicants with a wealth of life experience. Unlike many 'how to' books for standard entry courses, however, this book is written for the mature thinker. You will not find reference to the cost of a pint of beer anywhere in this book. Conversely, you will find, for instance, a detailed chapter on your future career; something which we rather hope is of concern to you.

The authors have made every effort to ensure that the information contained within is correct at the time of going to press. Neither the authors nor the editors can be held liable for any mistakes that may have been inadvertently overlooked in the preparation of this book. We take no responsibility for any external sources which we quote.

Why Medicine?

Medicine is the vocation of treating illness and preventing disease. The core of a degree in medicine is the study of the human body, in health and in disease. The range of subjects studied is exciting and demanding. In addition to the study of many different basic science 'ologies', students will also study public health, statistics, medical ethics and law, practical skills and gain an understanding of different cultures. Whilst absorbing this wealth of knowledge, students will be expected to gain understanding of the needs of patients and to communicate politely and effectively. Medicine is a fascinating and rapidly developing field and requires its doctors to undertake continuous professional and personal development. There are many career opportunities open to new doctors and a description of what happens after graduation is given in chapter 4. Whatever your chosen career, you will have an exciting and challenging time with highs and lows that are perhaps unsurpassed in most other careers.

Considering Medicine

Every year, some candidates apply to study medicine and yet have poorly considered reasons for making this choice. This, in turn, often leads (appropriately) to such candidates failing to gain entrance to medical school. Even worse, they often do not realise that their questionable motivations might cause concern.

In this chapter we outline the pros and cons of wanting to undertake medicine as a career. Some of the perspectives we present may seem harsh, but we believe they are all essential considerations. The chapter is written with two groups of people in mind. One group of readers are simply considering medicine as a career and would like to know more. The remainder, undoubtedly the vast majority, have already made a firm decision to study medicine and would like to know how to get in. Whichever you are, try at least to pretend that you have not yet made a firm decision to study medicine. The aim of the chapter is to challenge your motives for studying medicine such that you become more certain, or conversely that you realise you need to undertake more research.

If the following sounds a lot like you imagine a medical school interview to be, then you may well be right. However, this chapter is not concerned with how to answer questions at interview. The hope is that you will ask yourself similar questions in the context of making the right decision and hence maximise your chances of fulfilment. Many people are able to answer interview questions well but sometimes interviewers are left with the feeling that certain candidates have simply managed to convince themselves of what they are saying without holding any true underlying convictions. If your decision to study medicine is rational and honest not only are you more likely to obtain a place to study medicine but you are also much more likely to enjoy your chosen career!

Frankly speaking, perhaps you are applying to medical school now because you stormed into an inappropriate career on the basis of inadequate research. It would be unwise to make the same mistake again. Are you as convinced now as you were then? Are you insatiable and simply seeking yet another challenge? Do you hate exams? Answering yes to any of these questions does not disprove your suitability to study medicine, but should at least convince you that this life long commitment deserves serious consideration.

Also, are you being pushed or pulled into medicine? Some candidates are so disillusioned with their current careers and/or employers that they are reaching out for something (anything?), which will reduce the black hole developing in their soul. It may be that they are suited to medicine, but sometimes the 'push' seems to overwhelm any 'pull' so much as to make it almost invisible. It can be difficult for the candidates and their potential colleagues to determine suitability when it exists in a cloud of negativity.

Another common and potentially worrying reason for wanting to study medicine is a desire to please one's family. Personal satisfaction is not synonymous with parental pride. Arguably, there are merits to wanting to please one's family. For some people, this may be an incredibly strong driving force and may remain so for the rest of their life. Similarly, it would be rather ironic for someone to want to study medicine for entirely selfish reasons. It is hoped that medics care for other people, care for others' happiness and find reward in making those lives better. When a candidate's primary motivation is to please their family, concern may arise from the fact that this sentiment has often not forged long-term motivation, nor an ability to cope with stress, particularly when that family is no longer alive or supportive. In short, whilst a desire to please your family is honourable, is it enough to satisfy you and your patients for the rest of your life? If the answer is yes, then you should at least be aware that many interviewers might not empathise with this view.

Another classic and well publicised 'poor' reason for someone wanting to study medicine is that of 'wanting to make a difference'. Assuming that 'making a difference' means some bold and global act of nobility, this statement smacks of naivety and is also pretty inaccurate. Unique individuals in many walks of life make differences. A few doctors do 'make a difference' but most *good* doctors spend their time simply doing a good job within good guidelines, for patients who mostly have a narrow range of conditions within any given specialty. Medicine is not rocket science, and it's often not even interesting. Patients, however, are uniquely fascinating and the insight into their lives should be a privilege.

If making a difference for you means comforting a patient, earning the trust of a frightened child, or motivating a smoker to quit for the first time (not forgetting the vast majority of other patients who are not so moved), then making a difference may well be a very good reason to become a doctor. It is realism that is important. If you want to 'save lives' you should consider becoming a paramedic or going to a developing country. The usual aim of medicine is at best to prolong life, and improve its quality. Even then, these two aims can be frighteningly conflicting, but that ethical discussion is beyond the scope of this book. Your own ethical consideration is appropriate now, *before* you are confronted with a dying patient at 4am whose eyes remind you of those of your own grandmother.

Many people find themselves drawn to medicine following death or serious illness in their family. Some have witnessed wonderful care and view those doctors as role models. Others have witnessed unsatisfactory care and seek the opportunity to prevent another loved one from a similar misery. These experiences are valuable, and may in the future help that candidate to see 'the heart attack in bed 9' as a relative's beloved father. However, in isolation these experiences are anecdotal and biased. Your empathy for your loved one must surely cloud that for the doctor whose shoes you seek to fill.

It is possible to generalise common 'poor' reasons for choosing medicine, yet the 'right' reasons are unique to the individual. A reason which could be right for one person could be wrong for another. It would also be potentially damaging to attempt to give you 'a right answer' (not least because everyone reading this book might use it). If your reason(s) for wanting to study medicine are honest, realistic, framed by your skills, and supported with evidence (such as work experience), then you should be the very best person to articulate that personal desire.

Work Experience

Many candidates seem to think that gaining relevant work experience is entirely for a tick box at interview. Yet it is really the only way to even begin to make a decision about studying medicine; even then you might get it wrong. Those who view work experience as such a necessary chore are invariably preoccupied with spending time with Professor Brilliant of the Ultra-Brilliant Department of Brilliantologists. Whilst seeing this brilliant god in action may be fascinating, it is unlikely to be any more use in leading you to a humble and rational decision than could be gained by watching a documentary about the weirdest disease in the world on a less than reputable TV channel. You need to decide if you can be surrounded by sick and/or needy people. Beyond that, you need to decide if you want to care for them. As a doctor, dealing with patients and their myriad of problems will become your bread and butter, so you need to get a taste for it as early in the process as possible.

Do you gain delight from knowing that you did something with grace, irrespective of patients' thanks? Can you cope with sadness, hostility (not just from patients), anxiety, complaint and litigation? Are you able to cope with this by virtue of empathy and respect for yourself and others? Do you recognise your limitations? Many consumers of NHS resources are not sick in the conventional sense, but are you frustrated by their presence or empowered by the knowledge that they are still in need? It is human to dislike some people, and patients are no exception, but can you work for them professionally without losing your own fundamentally human qualities? It is impossible to answer these questions without spending some time with the types of people that you will be surrounded by as a doctor. Whilst extensive reading and familiarity with the system are useful, they are insufficient. The attitude of 'well my father is a doctor so I know everything there is to know about it' is fallible. How does this actually tell you how you will *feel*? Once qualified, even if you seek a specialty that has limited patient contact you must spend thousands of hours with patients before arriving in your professional comfort zone. It would be preferable that both you and your patients enjoy that transition period.

There are many ways of obtaining decent work experience. Not doing so is rarely excusable, and demonstrates a shallow interest in medicine and a lack of considered investment in your career choice. We have devoted a chapter to various aspects of work experience (see chapter 6).

Who are Tomorrow's Doctors?

The General Medical Council's education committee, which has responsibility in law for promoting high standards of medical education, have produced a series of publications (available online at: www.gmc-uk.org) relating to the future of medical education. It is recommended that you read *Tomorrow's Doctors* (1993), upon which so many graduate entry programmes have been closely designed. *Tomorrow's Doctors* made extensive recommendations on undergraduate medical education. Recommendations made in 2003, which replace those published in 1993, further identify the knowledge, skills, attitudes and behaviour expected of new graduates. The emphasis has moved from simply gaining knowledge (indeed, a reduction of the learning burden is recommended) to a greater inclusion of the other essential skills, attitudes and behaviour needed to interact with patients and colleagues.

Schools should ensure that only those who are fit to become doctors are allowed to enter medical school and therefore it stands to reason that they are looking for candidates who at least show the potential to achieve the proposed outcomes of *Tomorrow's Doctors*.

The duties of a doctor registered with the General Medical Council include:

> *'Make the care of your patient your first concern;*
> *Treat every patient politely and considerately;*
> *Respect patients' dignity and privacy;*
> *Listen to patients and respect their views;*
> *Give patients information in a way they can understand;*
> *Respect the rights of patients to be fully involved in decisions about their care;*
> *Keep your professional knowledge and skills up to date;*
> *Recognise the limits of your professional competence;*
> *Be honest and trustworthy;*
> *Respect and protect confidential information;*
> *Make sure that your personal beliefs do not prejudice your patients' care;*
> *Act quickly to protect patients from risk if you have good reason to believe that you or a colleague may not be fit to practise;*
> *Avoid abusing your position as a doctor; and*
> *Work with colleagues in the ways that best serve patients' interests.'*

Tomorrow's Doctors is the cornerstone guidance which has permitted medical schools to introduce new curricula that put the principles of professional practice, as set out in *'Good Medical Practice'* (including those above), at the centre of undergraduate education. Many recommendations are echoed in the medical school prospectuses.

It is often noted that doctors must have good communication skills. You should not have got this far without having some idea as to why that is important. But what is good communication? As for many skills, the guidance set out *Tomorrow's Doctors* provides a great insight into good communication, including:

' 23. Students must have opportunities to practise communicating in dif-
    ferent ways, including spoken, written and electronic methods. There
    should also be guidance about how to cope in difficult circumstances.
    Some examples are listed below.

    a. Breaking bad news.
    b. Dealing with difficult and violent patients.
    c. Communicating with people with mental illness, including cases
        where patients have special difficulties in sharing how they feel and
        think with doctors.
    d. Communicating with and treating patients with severe mental or
        physical disabilities.
    e. Helping vulnerable patients.'

Such detail *Tomorrow's Doctors* allows you to really think about whether you might have the necessary skills to be a good doctor, to consider your own experiences in context, and to go beyond a simple awareness that certain skills are important. The effect of this GMC guidance shows itself in most medical schools, at all stages from selection, to course design, to assessment.

Special Circumstances
Although special circumstances can relate to both undergraduates and graduates, issues surrounding age and children are more frequently raised within the latter group.

Age
The United Kingdom has an arguably healthy diversity of attitudes towards what is a suitable entry age. In the United States, medical students must hold a degree before they can enrol. In France, it is very unusual for medical students to be anything but school leavers; an attitude echoed throughout most of Europe.

It is difficult to discuss the advantages and disadvantages of being an older student without ostracising the younger candidate (as evidenced by the letters page of the popular medical student journal, 'The Student BMJ'). The statements below are simply generalisations; all students are unique and there are certainly many 'mature' students who are anything but mature. Since a 'mature' student is strictly one that is over 21 years of age, we have tried to use the term 'older' to mean mid to late thirties or so.

Many older students find that learning, particularly rote learning, is far more difficult than when they were in their early twenties. However, graduates have often acquired improved study methods and thus save themselves time because they learn from their own mistakes (for example they tend to spend less time colouring-in their notes). An individual's filing system is rarely something that does not improve over the years. Age and/or a previous degree enables the individual to identify more easily what they should be learning and to recognise and address deficits in their learning. Having said that, the chorus 'do we need to know this' is all too often bleated from the ranks of graduate students, and their 'maturity' often seems to vanish, perhaps due to some sort of herd immunity.

Older applicants usually have better communication and social skills in addition to greater life experience. Their ability to see the bigger picture, particularly in a clinical scenario, often surpasses that of their younger colleagues. They often have more financial security, and are likely to be free from the shackles of their previous degree's debt. Mature students have unique attitudes toward their younger colleagues, and vice versa. Some 'become young' again, whilst others maintain their previous lifestyles. How much an individual is liked by their medical seniors is as unique to that person's personality as for any student. Age, whilst sometimes used as a scapegoat, is unlikely to greatly influence the views of the other graduate students. The much older student may find that some doctors are highly sceptical of them (or threatened!), but this is undoubtedly balanced by the number who show greater respect.

Medical schools who offer graduate entry degree programmes necessarily value the mature student. Whilst there is no requirement for any newly qualified doctor to contribute to the NHS, it is inescapable that the older candidate is absolutely unable to contribute as much in years served as their younger counterpart potentially can. However, mature students tend to be happier doctors, quickly earn the respect of most of their colleagues, and the quality of their contribution may balance its reduced quantity. With its cost:benefit obsession, these issues are pertinent to the NHS and necessarily important to medical school committees. It can be argued that a quarter of a million pounds of tax payers' money, combined with approximately 10 years minimum training, should preclude those much over 40 years of age.

Schools are forbidden to discriminate on the basis of age and there is no legal requirement to work for the NHS. In practice, however, candidates over 40 years of age will have to be exceptional to be successful. Schools will feel that you have had more opportunity to gain valuable and varied work experience, and to have learnt more from those experiences. You must be realistic and enthusiastic about your career options, which are somewhat more limited than for younger students. It would not be disadvantageous to have undertaken further academic study.

It is worth consulting the prospectuses and the individual schools themselves to determine their latest policy and trends of upper age limits. Currently:

The University of Birmingham states that: 'We would find it hard to justify accepting any candidate over 40, since the minimum training period is 10 years.'

The University of Bristol states that: 'We do not have an upper age limit to medicine at Bristol ... and also be aware of the length of training following qualifying, as the average length of time from starting the programme and finally getting into the work/position wanted takes approximately 10 ten years.'

The University of Cambridge admissions manual states: 'There is no stated upper age limit for application to this course, but candidates should be able to give 25 years' service to the NHS after graduation. Work already undertaken in the NHS does count towards this total.'

The University of Leicester has no formal age limit and judges each application on its own merits, although the likely provision of service will be taken into account.

King's College London states that: 'Due to the length of professional training in medicine, it is unlikely for an applicant over 40 years of age to be considered and exceptional for an applicant over 45.'

The University of Liverpool states that: 'Because of the length of the course and the post-graduate training involved, we do not recommend anyone over the age of 40 applying.'

The University of Newcastle Upon Tyne states that: 'While we do not impose an upper age limit, applicants will be expected to demonstrate how, following graduation, they intend to provide significant service to the benefit of patients as a practising doctor'

The University of Nottingham states that: 'There is no upper age limit for admission to the GEM programme at the University of Nottingham.'

Oxford University states that: 'The graduate medicine technically does have an age limit but would strongly advise candidates who were 55+ that this may not be wise because of the length of the course.'

Queen Mary do not have an age limit.

The University of Southampton states that: 'There is no upper age limit for Medicine.'

St George's states that: 'We do not have an upper age limit. We advise candidates over the age of 45 to seriously consider the implications of starting such a demanding career at this age.'

University of Wales, Swansea states that: 'We do not impose an age limit or age restriction on this course. We simply give the same advice to every candidate regardless of their age to be aware of the length of time it takes to train before qualifying to work in this profession.'

The University of Warwick states no age limit: 'However we do advise that applicants over the age of 30 should carefully consider whether Medicine is the right option for them given the number of years it takes to fully qualify. This is advice, not an exclusion rule.'

Some medical schools without graduate entry programmes have an open attitude to the mature students. For instance, the University of East Anglia (UEA) in Norwich has accepted a 46 year old student - indeed, 57% of the first intake were mature students.

Children
Being a parent does not necessarily preclude you from getting through medical school, as mothers (and fathers) before you will testify. However, there are some important practical and emotional factors to consider.

Childcare options include nurseries, childminders, au pairs and nannies, with varying degrees of expense and flexibility. Financial support for childcare is made available to all full-time students by the Department for Education and Skills (DfES). In terms of nurseries, it may be necessary to secure a place more than a year in advance, which could present a difficult challenge when candidates may be informed of successful place offerings only months before the commencement of the course. Consider approaching private, council and university nurseries, in addition to the hospital nurseries, although the latter rarely offer places to non-NHS staff. The younger the child, the harder it can be to secure a place.

Depending on childcare arrangements, it may be difficult to put in many hours in at the hospital outside 9am to 5pm. However, it may be possible to negotiate different on-call schedules from those of fellow students. Similarly, some mothers have found that it is easier to secure weekend care for their child, so they may choose to study at the weekends.

Placements at far away district general hospitals also present a potential problem, although some schools are certainly prepared to take this into account for student parents. It is advisable to contact the medical schools directly to find out how far away clinical placements might be and the likelihood of receiving special consideration as a parent and carer.

Socially speaking, 'medical mums' are rarely found propping up the bar in the student union every night - or any night, for that matter. Balancing student life with a circle of mum and baby friends can be hard. Mothers' coffee mornings are a far cry from student life. A medical mum may feel that she and her child are missing out when friends are taking their babies to Aquatots and the like, but there are many mums who wish they had gone back to work.

Arguably, being a medical mum is no different to being a working mum, apart from the possibility of part-time work; something that a medical degree most certainly is not. A child should not have to miss out; there are plenty of activities at nursery and most mums feel able to make the most of weekends and holidays together. However, medical mums tend to have very well organised schedules, and have a stronger need than most to stick determinedly to their allocated study time.

Disability

Although dyslexia is the most common disability, students with a range of disabilities can successfully gain entry to medical school and complete the course.

Tomorrow's Doctors states: '... *students with a wide range of disabilities or health conditions can achieve the set standards of knowledge, skills, attitudes and behaviour. Each case is different and has to be viewed on its merits. The safety of the public must always take priority.'*

The newly qualified doctor with certain disabilities would find it impossible to carry out some of the clinical tasks normally associated with the first year of practice. For many years, the Medical Act has made special provision for doctors with a lasting physical disability, such that they can obtain alternative and relevant experience.

Attitudes toward graduate medical students

As with any fundamental change, some of your future medical colleagues will be less embracing of the newer styles of training. Whilst this scepticism will be less apparent by the time you are spending extensive amounts of time on the wards, it is likely to continue until the next phase of change in medical education. For example, some consultants view the requirement for only essential core knowledge as inappropriate, not least because they had to learn the intricacies of the

Krebs cycle (the bane of a medical student's biochemistry class) and want everyone else to, irrespective of whether it is relevant to patient care. They may also feel that the emphasis on personal development (sometimes rather derogatively referred to as 'fluff') is out of touch with the reality of a busy hospital.

These attitudes are directed at all medical courses that are quite rightly implementing the recommendations of *Tomorrow's Doctors*, but some doctors seem to associate such changes most closely with the graduate entry programmes. In addition to knowledge, a medical student needs to develop interpersonal skills, have maturity, and empathise with both patients and other staff. Where a doctor disputes this, it is probably because he does not possess those qualities himself.

One of the unspoken difficulties of being a mature medical student is the need to sometimes withstand adverse treatment from one's age-matched senior; often the challenge for a mature student is to conceal one's gall at such inappropriateness. Whilst most doctors will treat a mature medical student fairly, there are some senior doctors who have the capacity to be so improbably rude towards their juniors that it would make one's jaw drop. Unfortunately, the 'network' is such that it can take a Herculean bravery to defend oneself. Whilst this level of disrespect should not be directed towards any junior doctor or colleague, it is perhaps harder for a graduate to accept because in their pre-med life they have often been in a position of seniority.

The profession of medicine is a multitude of elements, and every rose has its thorn. It is difficult to cover all possible aspects of the profession, and even more difficult to do so honestly without inciting reaction. We have attempted to cover some essential features that you would be wise to contemplate.

Medical Schools

For each of the 14 schools offering graduate entry courses, you will find here a brief outline of the admission and selection details and statistics, course design, accommodation and contact details. We strongly recommend that you check the most current prospectuses and websites and confirm any information upon which you are dependent.

Gaining entry to graduate entry medicine presents every candidate with stiff competition and a diversity of choice. With any application process, being in possession of the most relevant and detailed information about that medical school confers considerable advantage and of course the power of choice. You would be surprised by the number of people who present to interview without showing any level of knowledge about the course for which they're applying. In this chapter, we have compiled core information that will help you to make quick sense of your choices. You must read the prospectuses in order to make a fully informed choice. There is simply insufficient space to detail all the information that you should know before making your application, and the information detailed here can only be correct at the time of writing.

Admission statistics and accommodation details relate to 2005 entry and should be used as a guide only.

Admission and Selection
Many candidates try to play the numbers game, and apply to those schools with the lowest ratio of applicants to places. Whilst we have included these numbers here, please note that, for instance, one school last year accepted

only candidates who held a first class degree. Instantly it can be seen that a simple ratio of applicants to places might not indicate an *easier* application procedure. It would be very difficult, if not impossible, to statistically determine which schools are 'the easiest' to get into. Similarly, candidates often comment on the variable difficulty of entrance exams. This makes little difference to your application; a difficult exam will have low marks *across the board* and vice versa; it is your relative position within the pack that matters. In fact, if you believe that many people might avoid a 'difficult' exam, applying to such schools could statistically advantage you! Degree class and subject not withstanding, you should aim for a school which you like, a course design and attitude which you like, then simply try your best. The time spent trying to work out which school is easiest to get into could instead be spent revising for an entrance exam or gaining further work experience.

The requirements listed here are those advertised at the time of writing. Please check individual prospectuses to confirm the requirements, and check schools' policies for special circumstances. Some schools have been known to lower their advertised requirements in light of other qualifications or experience. A satisfactory health declaration and a criminal record check are required prior to registration for all courses. See chapter 8 for details of entrance exams and chapter 9 for each school's interview procedures.

Standard Entry vs. Graduate Course
Accelerated graduate entry courses did not exist in the UK a decade ago, but already there are 14 graduate entry programmes. Although the majority of courses do not yet have a proven track record, there are no reasons for concern so far. Also, there is no reported disparity between arts and science graduates getting onto the courses and successfully graduating. The most notable differences of a graduate course are:

- *Shorter and highly intensive courses*
- *NHS bursary for years 2-4 to those eligible*
- *Greater emphasis on self directed learning*
- *Wider access*
- *Often there are no A-level or GCSE requirements*
- *A number of entrance exams*
- *Study alongside more similar age students*
- *Often less pre-clinical/clinical divide i.e. a more integrated course*

Website chat rooms are rife with suggestions that candidates should 'hedge their bets' by applying to standard entry courses in addition to the graduate entry courses. Although the ratio of applicants to places can appear to favour the standard entry courses, there are limited places for mature students so those statistics are not relevant and could be misleading. Also, for the few schools that will comment on the subject, they seem to imply that eligible graduates should apply to the graduate course. However, candidates are not penalised for applying to both courses, and their applications are treated independently. The exceptions to this rule are Swansea and Warwick, for the simple reason that they do not have a standard entry course; Oxford, which does not allow candidates to apply for both courses, and King's, whose graduate entry applicants are automatically considered for their standard entry course as well. For the most part, schools simply recommend that you apply to a school and course that is right for you.

Course Structure

Most of the graduate entry courses have an integrated course design, where clinical work is undertaken alongside academic study, as opposed to more traditional courses where the clinical years follow independently from pre-clinical study. There are a number of teaching methods associated with graduate courses, and these approaches are being phased into many standard courses. The balance between clinical exposure, problem-based learning tutorials, lectures and special study modules varies from one medical school to another. As graduate entry courses evolve the balance of learning tools will be frequently adjusted.

PBL

In problem-based learning (PBL), small groups of students look at the details of a patient's case, or problem. The students identify the likely problem(s) and use these issues to direct key areas in their learning. Self-directed learning thus relates the physiology, pharmacology, anatomy etc to the particular case. Patient contact and lectures are used to support this learning. In contrast to more traditional courses, subjects are not studied as academic stand-alone blocks, but in a continually developing and integrated nature. For some students this can seem daunting initially, but has the advantage that the rich tapestry of medicine is woven at an early stage.

Some schools' PBLs are simply chaired by a trained facilitator who does not necessarily have a scientific or medical background, whilst other schools' PBLs are tutored by a scientist or clinician.

CBL

Most schools use the term case-based learning (CBL) synonymously with PBL.

Self-directed Learning

PBL/CBL courses lend themselves to self-directed learning because it is invariably the students who are defining their learning objectives. Although such students are given support through e.g. lectures, these tend to be far fewer than on the traditional courses. Graduates are expected to be able to research and learn material by themselves, but students who prefer more lectures and direction may feel slightly overwhelmed. The biggest problem with self-directed learning seems to relate to insecurities about how *much* should be learnt and to what depth, as opposed to any inherent difficulty with independent study.

Amalgamation with standard course

Most, but not all, of the fast track graduate entry programmes at some stage merge with that medical school's concurrent standard medical course. Advantages of amalgamation are that you will follow a well-trodden route, with a potentially greater understanding of your role and requirements. Joining predominantly younger students is rarely a problem for either group, and will happen upon qualification anyway. However, a system that is unique to the graduate course can lead to novel and efficient schemes that allow greater flexibility.

Electives

An elective period is one of weeks or months in which the student can choose their own area of study, often abroad, in order to witness and become involved in an aspect of medicine they are particularly interested in or would not otherwise be exposed to. Most students travel to a specialist clinic or hospital. Due to the time constraints of the accelerated courses, some schools are unable to offer an elective period.

Formative and Summative Assessments

Although the assessment strategies for each school are not discussed here, it is useful to understand the terms when reading the prospectuses. Summative assessments are those exams which a student must pass in order to continue their training. Formative assessments often take the same form as the summative assessments but they are set for the students' benefit. Of course, a continuously poor performance in formative assessments should alert the student and staff to the risk of failure such that steps can be taken to raise the candidate's standard for the summative assessments.

Attachments and Firms

An 'attachment' refers to a period of time spent attached to a clinical setting, usually a particular department or an entire hospital. The time spent on that attachment is shared with other medical students and is usually dedicated to covering particular themes, for example the clinical attachment for surgery, or for specialties such as ear, nose and throat (ENT). In the UK, the term 'firm' has always been used historically in the clinical setting to refer to the team covering a particular ward, outpatient clinic or clinical section of department. It does not mean you have to arrive in a pinstriped suit.

Special Study Module (SSM)

In *Tomorrow's Doctors* the GMC recommended the introduction of Special Study Modules (SSM) to widen students' participation in projects or aspects of medicine that might ordinarily be slightly less common or inaccessible, or just to encourage students to take part in an aspect of medicine that is of their own choosing. Medical schools incorporate the SSM period into most years of the course. In some cases the SSM can compulsorily be a research project, while in the later clinical years SSMs can be non-clinical and explore disciplines on the periphery of medicine. To quote *Tomorrow's Doctors*, the SSM is an '... opportunitiy to study, for example, a language or to undertake a project related to literature or the history of medicine'.

Finance and Accomodation

The financial issues of studying on a graduate entry course are detailed in chapter 5.

Most schools can provide University or College accommodation in the first year. The availability of this accommodation to first year students is indicated below. Current price ranges are given here, and depend on facilities such as en suite, catered facilities, separate study and so forth.

Private accommodation prices indicated here are the average advertised prices on www.findaproperty.co.uk at the time of writing. Where possible, the prices have been given for one person, based on three sharing.

The University of Birmingham (B32) Medicine (Graduate Entry) (4 yrs) (A101)

First cohort 2002

Admission and Selection
- *Minimum 2:1 Honours degree in a life science discipline. Chemistry equivalent to grade C or better at A-level. In reality, only those with 1st class degree will be interviewed. Candidates must have been working in a medically related field within the last 2-3 years.*
- *662 applicants : 400 interviewed : 42 places*
- *Deferred entry is permitted.*
- *Applications from international students are not accepted.*
- *Interviews are held from October March.*

Course Structure
- *Year 1: PBL, predominantly self-directed learning.*
- *Year 2: Fewer PBLs. Partial amalgamation with the third-years on the five-year MBChB.*
- *Year 3 & ;4: Essentially full amalgamation with the five-year MBChB.*
- *8 week elective period*

Accommodation
- *University accommodation: 95% of first years can be accommodated, price range £290-540 pcm depending on facilities.*
- *Private accomodation: £354 pcm based on 2 sharing.*

Catchment Area
- *Very local - furthest is Wolverhampton.*

University population who are mature students : 11%

Contact

www.bham.ac.uk/
C.J.Lote@bham.ac.uk
0121 414 6888/6921/3481

University of Bristol (B78) Medicine
Graduate entry (4 years) (A101)

First cohort 2004

Admission and Selection

- *Minimum 2:1 in a bio-medical subject. BBB at A-level including Chemistry (unless included in degree). Candidates should consider at least 3 months' experience as a healthcare assistant or similar.*
- *554 applicants : 50 interviewed : 19 places*
- *Deferred entry is not permitted.*
- *Applications from international students are not accepted.*
- *Interviews are held from November - April.*

Course Structure

- *Condensed version of the 5 year MB ChB course with much amalgamtion between the two.*
- *Integration of clinical experience with core science and extensive tutorial group support.*
- *This is a traditional style of course, not problem based, with lectures, practicals, small-group teaching and supplemented by self-directed learning and illustrative clinical problems.*
- *10 week elective period*

Accommodation

- *Halls accommodation in first year: £125 pcm - £333 pcm depending on facilities.*
- *Private accommodation: £207 pcm based on 3 sharing.*

Catchment Area

- *Cheltenham, Swindon, Penzance, all of SE England*

University population who are mature students : 7%

Contact

    www.bristol.ac.uk

    admissions@bristol.ac.uk

    0117 928 7679

University of Cambridge (C05)
Cambridge Graduate Course in Medicine (A101)

First cohort 2001

Admission and Selection

- *Minimum 2:1 degree or equivalent, in any discipline, who also satisfy the pre-medical requirements.*
- *Candidates must complete the UCAS application form, the Cambridge Application Form and a separate application form for the Graduate Course in Medicine.*
- *Applicants are not required to sit the BMAT unless they wish to use a successful result as part of their pre-medical requirements.*
- *Applicants to the graduate course may also apply to Oxford University.*
- *201 applicants : 75 interviewed : 20 places*
- *Deferred entry is not permitted.*
- *Applications from international students are not accepted.*
- *Interviews are held in the last week of November*

Course Structure

- *First 4.5 terms: fully amalgamated with conventional course, with lectures and tutorials. Clinical attachments take place during the normal university vacations.*
- *After 4.5 terms, the clinical component of the graduate course is in part amalgamated with the conventional clinical course. The remainder combines hospital-based and community-based clinical learning.*
- *The main clinical base for the Cambridge Graduate Course (CGC) is in Bury St Edmunds.*
- *Throughout: additional small group work sessions, facilitated by a senior clinician from the West Suffolk Hospital.*
- *No opportunity for a standard elective.*

Accomodation

- *There are no college fees for this course.*
- *College accommodation available for all 3 years at about £80 - £90 per week*
- *Private accommodation: £304 pcm based on 3 sharing*

Catchment Area

- *Bury St Edmunds, Cambridge, Peterborough, Papworth*

University population who are mature students : 4%

Contact

www.cam.ac.uk/admissions/undergraduate
admissions@cam.ac.uk
01223 333 308

King's College London (University of London) (K60) Graduate/Professional Entry Programme (Medicine) (A102)

First cohort 2004

Admission and Selection

- *Minimum 2:1 honours degree in any subject or 2:2 honours degree with a post-graduate degree or a Diploma of Higher Education in Nursing at a pass, with at least 2 years post-qualification nursing work experience.*
- *Health service professionals without an honours degree, but with appropriate post-qualification experience, may be considered.*
- *Candidates are called to interview on the basis of their MSAT result (91st centile, ~70% in 2005).*
- *1100 applicants : 130 interviewed: 24 places*
- *Deferred entry is permitted.*
- *Applications from international students are accepted.*
- *Interviews are held in February & March.*
- *Candidates are given automatic consideration for the standard 5 year course.*

Course Structure

- *Throughout the course there is full integration of science and clinical teaching.*
- *Year 1: Separate teaching for the graduate course, at the Guy's Campus. CBL & PBL with clinician or scientist, patient contact, small groups, clinical and practical.*
- *Years 2-4: Students join those of the other MB BS streams for a common course, taught together in small groups of 2 to 8 students, attached to clinically active teams in 'firms'.*
- *8 week elective period.*

Accomodation
- *First year accommodation £250-£333 pcm depending on facilities*
- *Private accommodation: £960 pcm based on 2 sharing (London SE1 postcode)*

Catchment Area
- *South London and locations throughout SE England, includes Kent and Medway*

University population who are mature students : 18%

Contact
> www.kcl.ac.uk
> gktadmissions@kcl.ac.uk
> 020 7848 6501/6502

University of Leicester (L34)
Medicine (4 years) (A101)

First cohort 2002

Admission and Selection

- *2:1 Honours degree in a Health Science or related discipline.*
- *A-level and GCSE examinations are not considered.*
- *Degrees considered include Health Sciences, Health Studies, Nursing, Physiotherapy, Optometry, Psychology, Radiography, Podiatry, Mental Health, Occupational Health, Midwifery.*
- *Candidates can apply to only Leicester or Warwick.*
- *500 applicants : 100 interviewed: 64 places*
- *Deferred entry is not permitted.*
- *Applications from international students are not accepted.*
- *Interviews are held in November - March.*

Course Structure

- *Condensed version of 5-year course.*
- *Integrated clinical and medical science throughout.*
- *Small groups, clinically related problems, a few lectures.*
- *Year 1: Separate course for graduate entry. PBL with clinical tutor.*
- *Year 2-4: fully amalgamated with standard entry course.*
- *There is the opportunity for an elective period of study.*

Accomodation

- *College accommodation guaranteed in first year £238 - £468 pcm depending on size and catering.*
- *Private accomodation: £184 pcm based on 3 sharing*

Catchment area

- *Furthest placements are: Kettering, Boston, Peterborough*

University population who are mature students : 12%

Contact

www.le.ac.uk/sm/le

med-admis@le.ac.uk

0116 252 2969/2963

The University of Liverpool (L41)
Medicine (Graduate Entry) (A101)

First cohort 2003

Admission and Selection
- *Minimum 2:1 in a Biomedical/Health Science degree plus a minimum of CCC at A-level including Biology and Chemistry.*
- *GCSEs in English and Maths (grade A or B) are also required.*
- *Applications should also submit a CV to the Admissions Tutor.*
- *650 applicants : 92 interviewed : 32 places*
- *Deferred entry is not permitted.*
- *Applications from international students are not accepted.*
- *Interviews are held in February or March.*

Course Structure
- *Year 1: Condensed version of years one and two of the 5 five-year programme. PBLs, some lectures, early clinical contact.*
- *Year 2 - 4: Full amalgamation with years 3-5 of standard course, with PBLs and clinical sessions.*
- *5 week elective period*

Accomodation
- *College first year accommodation provided at £300-4300 pcm depending on facilities*
- *Private accomodation: £328 pcm based on 2 sharing*

Catchment Area
- *Furthest are: Barrow-in-Furness, Kendal, Lancaster*

University population who are mature students : 18%

Contact
> www.liv.ac.uk
> mbchb@liv.ac.uk
> ugrecruitment@liv.ac.uk
> 0151 794 2000
> 0151 706 4266

University of Newcastle Upon Tyne (N21)
Medicine (Accelerated Programme, Graduate Entry) (A101)

First cohort 2002

Admission and Selection
- *Minimum 2:1 Honours degree in any discipline or be a practising health professional with a post-registration qualification.*
- *Applicants are expected to show evidence of academic endeavour within the last 2-3 years.*
- *1000 applicants : 200 interviewed : 25 places*
- *Deferred entry is permitted.*
- *Applications from international students are not accepted.*
- *Interviews are held in November - March.*

Course Structure
- *Year 1: Independent from standard course. Integrated clinical and core science. CBLs are with a senior medical tutor.*
- *Year 2-4: Full amalgamation with 5 year course.*
- *8 week elective period*

Accomodation
- *Probable college accommodation in first year; £150 - £300 pcm depending on facilities.*
- *Private accomodation: £252 pcm based on 3 sharing*

Catchment Area
- *Tyne, Weir, Northumbria, Tees, Middlesborough*

University population who are mature students : 9%

Contact
www.ncl.ac.uk/undergraduate/course/A101
Medic.ugadmin@ncl.ac.uk
0191 2227005

The University of Nottingham (N84)
Medicine (Graduate Entry) (A101)

First year course ran: 2003

Admission and Selection

- *2:2 degree in any subject and a competitive score (62% in 2005) in the GAM-SAT examination.*
- *1100 applicants : 200-250 interviewed : 90 places*
- *Deferred entry is not permitted.*
- *Applications from international students are not accepted.*
- *Interviews are held in March - April .*

Course Structure

- *First 18 months: based in a purpose-built medical school building on the Derby City Hospital campus. PBL with a trained facilitator, early clinical experience, small-group teaching, lectures and demonstrations.*
- *18 months - 4 years: Full amalgamation with the five-year course with the same modules/attachments in a variety of clinical sites in the East Midlands.*
- *6 week elective period*

Accomodation

- *College accommodation in first year £218 - £358 pcm depending on facilities*
- *Private accommodation: £193 pcm Derby, based on 3 sharing*

Catchment Area

- *Trent area, Derby, Nottingham, Lincoln, Mansfield*

University population who are mature students : 6%

Contact

www.nottingham.ac.uk

gem@nottingham.ac.uk

01332 724622

Oxford University (O33)
Medicine (Fast-track, Graduate Entry only) (A101)

First cohort 2001

Admission and Selection
- *Minimum 2:1 degree in a bioscience or chemistry degree.*
- *Candidates must complete the UCAS application form, the Oxford Application Form including a short statement and 3 references.*
- *Shortlisting for interview is based on a 2 hour written test. Applicants to the graduate course may also apply to Cambridge.*
- *250 applicants : 90 interviewed : 30 places*
- *Deferred entry might be permitted.*
- *Applications from international students are accepted.*
- *Interviews are held in December.*

Course Structure
- *Year 1 & 2: Science taught within a clinical context (with a greater clinical emphasis in year 2). Problem-oriented seminars with specialist tutors, held after independent study of that topic. Very few lectures and highly self-directed, supported by college tutorials of two or three students.*
- *Years 3&4: Full amalgamation with standard entry course.*
- *10 week elective and other opportunities to go abroad.*

Accomodation
- *College accommodation: ~ £350 pcm*
- *Private accommodation: £601 pcm based on 3 sharing*

Catchment Area
- *Mostly local, includes: Milton Keynes, Banbury, Northampton, Reading, High Wycombe*

University population who are mature students : 4%

Contact

> bmra.pharm.ox.ac.uk
> undergraduate.admissions@admin.ox.ac.uk
> 01865 270212

Queen Mary, University of London (Q50)
Medicine (Graduate Entry) (A101)

First Cohort 2003

Admission and Selection

- *2:1 honours in a science or health related degree. Applicants will be invited to interview on the basis of their MSAT (86th centile, ~68% in 2005) result & UCAS and academic. 10 places are reserved for Queen Mary's Biomedical Sciences graduates and other medically-related courses at Queen Mary.*
- *1000 applicants : 120 interviewed : 40 places (note above reservation)*
- *Deferred entry is not permitted.*
- *Applications from international students are accepted.*
- *Interviews are held in March.*

Course Structure

- *Year 1: The course runs jointly with City University as a multi-professional course, where medical students join an equal number of graduates who are on accelerated courses leading to qualifications in nursing and in other professions allied to medicine. PBL*
- *Year 2: PBL and continued inter-professional learning.*
- *Year 3 & 4: Significant amalgamation with standard programme.*
- *12 week elective period*

Accomodation

- *First year accomodation £380 pcm at the Barts site*
- *Private accommodation: £614 pcm based on 3 sharing*

Catchment Area

- *Furthest are: Southend, Chelmsford*

Universitypopulation who are mature students : 21%

Contact
020 7601 7603
www.qmul.ac.uk
gepmedicine@qmul.ac.uk

University of Southampton (S27)
Medicine Graduate entry (4 year) (A101)

First Cohort 2004

Admission and Selection
- *2.1 honours degree, grade C or better at GCSE in English, Mathematics and Science, A-Level in Chemistry, or passes in Biology and Chemistry at AS-Level, or equivalent.*
- *Graduate applicants are not interviewed.*
- *1300 applicants : 0 interviewed: 40 places*
- *Deferred entry is permitted.*
- *Applications from international students are accepted.*
- *Interviews are held in December - March.*

Course Structure
- *Years 1 & 2: Small group work structured around clinical topics. Substantial clinical experience, and amalgamation with the 5 year programme for some lectures and practicals.*
- *Years 3 & 4: Similar programme to 3rd and 5th years of the 5 year programme.*
- *No opportunity for electives*

Accomodation
- *First year guaranteed; £260 - 555 pcm depending on facilities*
- *Private accommodation: £257 pcm based on 3 sharing*

Catchment Area
- *Includes: Portsmouth, Winchester, Southampton, Salisbury*

University population who are mature students : Data not available

Contact

    www.som.soton.ac.uk

    bmadmissions@soton.ac.uk

    023 8059 4408

St George's Hospital Medical School
(University of London) (S49)
Medicine (4-year Graduate Entry) (A101)

First Cohort 2000

Admission and Selection
- *2:2 honours degree in any discipline or a higher degree such as MSc, MA, MPhil or PhD. Candidates will be called to interview on the basis of their GAMSAT result.*
- *1500 applicants : 175 interviewed: 70 places*
- *Deferred entry is permitted.*
- *Applications from international students are not accepted.*
- *Interviews are held in the last week of March to the start of April.*

Course Structure
- *Year 1 & 2: PBL with trained facilitators, lectures, clinical skills. Integration of clinical teaching and core science.*
- *Year 3 & 4: Clinical attachments, independent of standard entry course.*
- *10 week elective.*

Accomodation
- *First year college accommodation provided at £260 pcm*
- *Private accommodation: £430 pcm based on 3 sharing*

Catchment Area
- *Mostly SW Thames region, but can be as far as:*
  Liverpool, Isle of Wight, Plymouth, Yeovil, Darlington

University population who are mature students : 30%

Contact

www.sgul.ac.uk

gep@sghms.ac.uk

020 8725 5201

University of Wales Swansea (S93)
Medicine (A101)

First Cohort 2004. No standard entry course.

Admission and Selection

- *2:1 in any degree. Candidates are selection for interview purely on the basis of the UCAS form. After interview, candidates will be selected on the basis of:*
- *UCAS form and overall academic ability (20%)*
- *GAMSAT Score (20%)*
- *Interview Performance (60%)*
- *Swansea only offers a graduate-entry programme.*
- *500 applicants : 175 interviewed: 70 places*
- *Deferred entry is not permitted.*
- *Applications from international students are not accepted.*
- *Interviews are held February.*

Course Structure

- *Years 1 & 2: Equivalent programme of study to the first 3 years of the Cardiff medical course. CBL. Integration of science and clinical medicine throughout.*
- *Years 3 & 4: Clinical training with teaching.*
- *6-8 weeks Elective*

Accomodation

- *First year college accommodation: £230 pcm*
- *Private accomodation: £195 pcm*

Catchment Area

- *All-Wales Clinical Training Rotation. The furthest are: Bangor, Wrexham*

University student population who are mature students : 16%

Contact

www.gemedicine.swan.ac.uk
medicine@swansea.ac.uk
01792 513400

The University of Warwick (W20)
Medicine MBChB (A101)

First Cohort 2000. No standard entry course.

Admission and Selection

- *2:1 degree in the biological sciences or related discipline or 2:2 with appropriate PhD.*
- *Candidates must complete a supplementary application form by 1st December.*
- *Candidates are called to interview on the basis of their MSAT result and UCAS form.*
- *Warwick only offers a graduate-entry programme. Candidates can only apply to the Leicester or Warwick programme.*
- *900 applicants : 350 interviewed: 164 places*
- *Deferred entry is not permitted.*
- *Applications from international students are accepted.*
- *Interviews are held February onwards.*

Course Structure

- *The course is a condensed version of the 5 year course at Leicester and removes those elements which graduates in the biological sciences are expected to have studied in depth.*
- *Year 1 & 2: Some lectures video linked to those of the Leicester standard course, small group work and early clinical experience.*
- *Year 3 & 4: Full amalgamation with Leicester 5 year course, with 8 week rotations.*
- *6 week elective period*

Accomodation
- *First year accommodation £216 - £300 (mostly off campus) depending on facilities.*
- *Private accommodation: £255 pcm based on 3 sharing*

Catchment Area
- *Clinical attachments are across all sites utilised by the Warwick Medical School: UHCW NHS Trust (Walsgrave), George Eliot (Nuneaton), The Alexandra Hospital Redditch, Warwick Hospital.*

University population who are mature students : 12%

Contact
med-admis@warwick.ac.uk
024 765 28101
024 765 74394
024 765 73813

A Medical Career

You're considering graduate entry medicine. You're currently focussing on how to get *in*. It may not seem to be such an immediate concern but it's just as important to think about what happens once you get *out* . . .

What does happen after you finish your training? Well, put simply, *more* training! Medicine offers a multitude of postgraduate career paths but none of them are quick, and some of them can take a very long time to complete. Whichever path you follow, you will be required to continue learning whilst you work by pursuing specialist training, continuing professional development programmes, and by taking further examinations. Keep in mind that this information applies whether you have graduated from a standard entry course or from a graduate entry course.

Whatever your long-term choices may be, the mechanics of initial postgraduate employment and training will be the same for all newly qualified doctors. When you graduate you will be allowed to use the courtesy title 'doctor' and you will be granted provisional registration as a medical practitioner with the statutory regulatory body, the General Medical Council (GMC). The vast majority of UK medical graduates will end up working for the NHS in one way or another so postgraduate medical training in the UK is predominantly geared toward meeting the medical workforce needs of the NHS and is therefore very closely tied to it.

There has been something of an assumption made in the past that medics from graduate-entry courses are GPs in the making. The assumption seems to follow the logic that graduate students are older and therefore wish to qualify more quickly. This is often not the case, but general practice is one of the quickest routes to full professional qualification. There are no career options that are closed to doctors from graduate-entry courses but, in reality, the longest, most specialised training programmes could prove difficult to get into (certain surgical specialties may take over ten years from graduation to completion). However, graduate-entry medicine thrives on its ability to challenge preconceptions, so go on - be a neurosurgeon if you want to!

The career goal of most doctors is to be either a senior hospital doctor ('Consultant') or a general practitioner ('GP principal'). Both of these are fully-qualified, independent medical practitioners who are ultimately responsible for the patients in their care. The length and type of training involved varies for different specialties, whilst general practice has its own training requirements. There are also a number of other possible careers both within and outside the NHS, some of which we will cover in a little more detail later. They include:

- *Other roles within the NHS*
- *Academic medicine*
- *Forensic medicine*
- *Armed services*
- *Public health*
- *Private practice*
- *Other non-NHS roles:*
  occupational health; industrial medicine; sports medicine.

Hospital specialty training and general practice training
The term 'junior doctor' covers all grades of hospital doctor before

reaching the position of Consultant. Progress through postgraduate training is supervised by local Postgraduate Deans. All the UK Deaneries are managed through the Conference of Postgraduate Medical Deans (COPMeD). Each Deanery is an umbrella for numerous Foundation Schools which manage the placement of new graduates in their respective hospitals. The way in which newly qualified junior doctors are trained and employed is undergoing a radical overhaul as part of a lengthy national review of all medical training by the UK Department of Health, known as *Modernising Medical Careers* (MMC).

Medical graduates will begin with a two-year Foundation Programme. This new concept, piloted in 2004 and implemented nationally from 2005, consists of general 'on the job' clinical training. It is designed to form a link between medical school teaching and higher training for hospital specialties or general practice. It comprises a series of placements in a variety of specialties and healthcare settings. Applications and appointments for the Foundation Programme are made in the autumn of the final year at medical school, but the precise nature of the application process is changing each year. The Government's stated aim is that the Foundation Programme will provide a much more structured approach to a new doctor's first two years of work. It will emphasise continued learning, with a specified range of outcome objectives, especially in the achievement of core clinical competencies. At the time of writing, the finer details of how this will work in practice are not fully defined but by the time you graduate it should be well and truly established.

The first year of the foundation programme (F1) replaces the former pre-registration house officer year (PRHO; sometimes referred to as junior house officer). This year is spent in approved, supervised posts and must include practical experience in both medicine and surgery. There may be two posts, each of six months' duration but it is more likely that F1 will comprise three four-month rotations, with the additional placement spent working in a different field, such as general practice.

Full registration with the GMC will be granted after completion of F1. The second foundation year (F2) is intended to be flexible. In essence it will be the equivalent of the first year of what is known as a Senior House Officer (SHO), as explained later. For those with a definite career path in mind, F2 posts could be arranged to contribute to that objective but the postgraduate deaneries are also keen to promote the idea that doctors may use F2 to expand their range of clinical experience. It has been proposed that short 'taster' rotations (especially in more unusual specialties) lasting just a few weeks could be interspersed between longer, more traditional posts. Some would argue that this is essentially just a way of promoting and recruiting for the less popular specialties.

The concept of attaining clinical competency objectives will continue from F1 into F2. In particular, the F2 competencies will relate to the recognition and management of seriously ill patients. It is possible that many postgraduate deaneries may make a rotation in Accident and Emergency medicine ('A&E') a required part of F2 for all doctors. Some deaneries are developing integrated foundation programmes, such that new graduates may apply for a fixed, two-year, F1+F2 rotation. Many of these two-year programmes have been designed with broad clinical specialties in mind so that new doctors may follow their interests. For example, an aspiring surgeon may choose to apply for a programme which incorporates more experience in surgical posts.

The two-year foundation appointments should allow participants to roughly plan where they will be living for the first two years of their professional life since the F1 and F2 posts are confined to those available within a specified geographical area served by its Foundation Schools. However, some of these areas are very large. For example, the

South West Thames Foundation School extends from South West London as far as Cornwall and includes every area in between (as detailed on the London Deanery website: www.londondeanery.ac.uk). To find out where you could work as an F1/F2, based on geographical region, go to the COPMeD website listed at the end of this chapter.

After the foundation programme, doctors will move into more specialised training posts, gaining further clinical experience in their chosen field and taking progressively more responsibility for patient care. The specialist training posts that follow the Foundation Programme and the nature of the career progression involved is also under review. Although the titles, job descriptions and the exact balance between service provision (i.e. 'on the ward' work) and training may change slightly, the overall duration of the training is unlikely to change all that much.

There are presently two grades for hospital doctors in training: Senior House Officer (SHO) and Specialist Registrar (SpR). Although there is no specified duration one should spend as an SHO, traditionally doctors have generally spent two to three years in SHO posts (usually of six months duration each), gaining broad experience of specialties relevant to their chosen career. This is referred to as 'basic specialist training'. Following this, appointment to SpR posts is by open competition. SpR posts are approved programmes, lasting five years or longer, which provide 'higher specialist training', leading to full qualification as a Consultant in the doctor's chosen specialty. One must then apply against open competition for a Consultant job. Each doctor entering higher specialist training is allocated a national training number (NTN; also referred to as a 'Calman number' after the Calman Report which led to the last re-organisation of medical training). The individually assigned number allows the Postgraduate Deans to track the progress of each doctor in specialist training.

Under MMC, the intention is that these grades (and possibly the traditional titles associated with them) will be phased out by 2007, in time for the first cohort of doctors completing the Foundation Programme to enter the new grade. SHO and SpR will be replaced by a single 'run-through' specialist training grade that would follow on from the end of F2 and ultimately lead to eligibility for Consultant or GP principal posts. The general description *Integrated Training* is being used at present but precisely what these posts will be called and how they will operate is presently unknown. The concept of competency-based assessment will also be introduced across higher specialty training as well as the foundation programme.

Clearly, the new approach will have an impact upon the career choices of new doctors as the decision about which specialty to follow will have to be made somewhat earlier than under the old system. Work is ongoing to develop integrated training posts that are broad-based and will minimise pressure on those doctors who do not have a particular specialty in mind as they leave the Foundation Programme. Proposals have been put forward that specialties which are likely to have significant overlap in the early stages of integrated training should develop common pathways for the first half of the grade. For example, there may be an initial common training pathway for all the surgical specialties and the same principle could be applied to other related specialties such as emergency medicine, anaesthesia and intensive care. There is also an acknowledgement that increased careers advice and support should be made available.

From September 2005 there is also a significant statutory administrative change to postgraduate medical training (see Fig. 1 for structure). For the first time, all postgraduate certification, whether for general practice or hospital specialties, will be brought together under one statutory awarding body, the *Postgraduate Medical Training and Education Board*

(PMETB). The current *Certificate of Prescribed Experience* (for general practice), awarded by the *Joint Committee on Postgraduate Training for General Practice* (JCPTGP), and the *Certificate of Completion of Specialist Training* (for hospital specialties), awarded by the *Specialist Training Authority* (STA), will be replaced by a common *Certificate of Completion of Training* (CCT). The award of a CCT is significant in that it allows a doctor to be included on the GMC's specialist register, which is required before a doctor can be appointed to a Consultant post within the NHS.

Training for general practice is slightly different to that for hospital specialists. Doctors who have completed their PRHO year are currently required to spend two years in SHO posts and one year as a GP registrar. It should be noted, however, that the JCPTGP, the authority with responsibility for the approval of GP training until PMETB goes live in September 2005, currently recommends that doctors who wish to be licensed to work as GPs in the NHS should plan to undertake a full three-year GP training programme *following* successful completion of their two-year Foundation Programme. This will essentially add another year to the duration of GP training.

Although there is a lot of uncertainty surrounding postgraduate training, what is unlikely to change in any way will be the requirement to study for (and pass) further professional examinations in your chosen specialty.

Postgraduate qualifications

There are a multitude of postgraduate professional qualifications, most of which take the form of *membership* or *fellowship* of the medical royal college relevant to a doctor's chosen specialty. This can be more than a little confusing. The reasons behind the different titles are mostly due to history and tradition and do not imply any difference in the seniority of the qualifications. The examinations for these qualifications tend to come in two parts and, under the current system, the first part is generally taken during the SHO years and may be an entry requirement for an SpR post. The second part is generally taken during the later stages of the SpR years and may be required in order to qualify for a certificate of completion of specialist training and entry onto the GMC specialist register. For example, to practice as a consultant surgeon one must have passed the fellowship of the Royal College of Surgeons, hence the postnominal 'FRCS' after a surgeon's name.

A full description of all the different medical royal colleges is beyond the scope of this chapter but each royal college has its own website and these usually offer information that covers in some detail the career paths which relate to their specialties and the qualifications they offer. With the establishment of the PMETB the medical royal colleges no longer have a formal role in the regulation of specialist training and appointments but they will undoubtedly continue to have significant influence in an advisory capacity.

Developing an understanding of research methodology is a part of specialist training and many doctors choose to complete a research diploma or higher degree, for example PhD or MD, in the midst of their SpR years. This is not a formal requirement for entry to a Specialist Registrar training programme or for subsequent appointment to a Consultant post, but for those specialties where competition for higher training posts is fierce you could be forgiven for believing that it was compulsory! It will be up to the PMETB, in association with the relevant medical royal college, to decide whether time spent in research posts should count towards specialist training.

Academic Medicine

Academic medicine is unique within the roles of medics. It entails the dual commitment of clinical work and academic research. Perhaps the two skills it demands most are grovelling for research funding and the art of juggling. Academic medicine has long been seen as under-resourced and the UK currently has a significant shortfall of medical academics. Clearly this has implications for future medical research and training so the development of a structured career path for medical academics is an integral part of MMC.

A recent report from an MMC sub-committee looking at the future of academic medicine (the 'Walport' report) has proposed that that there should be a dedicated academic medicine F2 year which will allow new doctors who are interested in research and teaching careers to begin to develop these interests at an early stage. Alternatively, a four-month academic rotation may be offered as one of the posts within the F2 year for those who wish to explore the possibility of a career in academic medicine. Similarly, there will eventually be integrated training programmes that set out clear training pathways for those doctors wishing to pursue an academic career.

Academic medics are usually employed by their parent University or College and hold honorary clinical posts with local NHS organisations, although some academics may be employed jointly by a university and the NHS. Most medical academics provide clinical services to patients through the NHS as well as teach medical students and undertake research. Lecturers are usually given honorary Registrar posts, and Senior Lecturers, Readers and Professors hold honorary Consultant posts appropriate to their specialist qualifications. Many junior posts are for fixed terms but senior academic positions can be for longer fixed terms (e.g. 5 years), tenured or on permanent appointments. However, academic medicine is not necessarily the most secure position because research funding must be constantly sought and renewed, and can range from as little as 1 year of funding up to 10 years. Medically qualified staff may also be employed by academic institutions to carry out non-clinical teaching and research but they are employed under the same terms as non-medically qualified university teachers, not as clinical academics.

Other hospital posts within the NHS

As well as the standard training posts described above, you may also hear a vast and confusing number of other job titles. Many such titles (Clinical Fellow, Research Fellow, Middle Grade and Trust Clinician to name but a few) are associated with non-standard posts that have been created by individual hospital trusts around the UK. Some of these posts may incorporate a training component that is recognised and counted towards specialist qualification by the relevant royal colleges, but many do not. Some doctors may choose to take one of these posts (such as a clinical teaching or research post) to gain addition professional experience in a particular area. Others may spend time in such a post as a 'stop-gap' between basic and higher specialist training. This bottle-neck between SHO and SpR is something which the new integrated specialist training programmes are intended to relieve.

Alongside the training posts for junior doctors there are also a number of specific non-training posts for doctors who prefer to work in hospitals but who do not wish, or are not able, to become Consultants. These are permanent posts and they are purely concerned with service provision; there is no allocated training component to these roles so they can be something of a dead-end as far as further career progression is concerned. These are the standard NHS grades for hospital doctors other than juniors in training and Consultants:

Staff grade doctors have an intermediate level of clinical responsibility, delegated to them by the Consultants to whom they are responsible; they do not have continuous 24-hour responsibility for patients in the way that Consultants do. Full GMC registration and at least three years experience at SHO grade, including time in the relevant specialty, are needed for these positions. Most doctors who enter this grade will stay there for the rest of their careers and the opportunities to subsequently progress to other grades can be very limited.

Associate Specialists, unlike staff grade doctors, are regarded as senior hospital doctors although they are technically responsible to a named Consultant. Associate specialist appointments are often 'one-off' posts created for individual experienced doctors who have, for some reason, not been able to achieve Consultant status. To be eligible, doctors must have at least ten years' postgraduate experience, including time in registrar or staff grade posts, with at least two years in the appropriate specialty. Associate specialists have contracts similar to Consultants and their working arrangements generally mirror those of their Consultant colleagues rather than those of the junior doctors.

There are also a number of hospital-based roles for qualified general practitioners within the NHS system. Some GPs appreciate the additional clinical experience and the challenge of spending some of their time in a specialist area in which they have an interest. These roles, termed *Clinical Assistant* or *Hospital Practitioner,* are often part-time and the doctors who undertake them work as part of a medical team, led by a Consultant. They are usually GP principals who have experience in the relevant specialty and they often hold an appropriate specialist diploma.

Salaries

Doctors working for the NHS are paid in line with the recommendations of the Doctors and Dentists Review Body (DDRB). To give you a feel for the numbers, these are the basic salaries, by grade, for NHS hospital doctors in England in 2005. F1/F2 salaries are not denoted below because they vary slightly from the House Officer salary due to the junior doctor's contractual obligation to the European Working Time Directive (EWTD):

Grade	Basic salary (£/pa)
Junior hospital doctors	
House Officer	19,703 - 22,240
Senior House Officer	24,587 - 34,477
Specialist Registrar	27,483 - 41,733
Senior hospital doctors	
Consultant (new contract)	67 133 - 90 849
Additional clinical excellence awards and discretionary points may also be paid:	
Local	2 702 - 32 424
National	32 424 - 69 261
Non-Consultant career grades	
Staff Grade	30 808 - 43 871
Inc. additional discretionary points	45 946 - 58 562
Associate Specialist	34 158 - 61 935
Inc. additional discretionary points	63 703 - 75,233

If you think that these figures look a little low, especially in the early years, do bear in mind that these are only *basic* salaries and that an additional banding system is in operation for junior doctors. The pay-bands take account of hours worked above the nominal 40 hours per week, the type of working pattern (shifts), the frequency of any additional duties and the unsocial nature of the hours worked. The total salary comprises the full base salary to which a supplement is then added. The pay-bands are also subject to review by the DDRB and they currently range from supplements of 20% up to 100% of basic pay for full-time doctors. A number of awards may also be made to Consultants and other career grade doctors in addition to their basic salaries.

Other medical careers

A full review of all the medical career options is beyond the scope of this introduction. Many paths such as occupational health or work for the Home Office, the police or the prison service develop after doctors have undertaken initial training posts within NHS hospitals.

Public health medicine is a unique specialty that has responsibility for disease prevention and the promotion of health on a population basis. It requires a sound knowledge of both clinical practice and the specialist areas of epidemiology, medical statistics and social sciences. Public health medicine therefore has its own specific career pathway which doctors usually enter after several years of normal professional training within the NHS.

Medicine in the armed forces is another specialist area in its own right. Military medical careers parallel their civilian counterparts in that GMC registration is still required and higher specialist training and royal college qualifications are also an integral part of career progression. Alongside this there is a requirement to undertake further military training as a commissioned officer with the relevant service. A benefit to armed services medical training is the considerable financial support received whilst a medical student (commencing salary of approximately £15,000 with fees and maintenance paid) and subsidised housing while in service. There is currently a significant shortfall of doctors in the defence medical services. Further information may be found under the careers sections of the websites of the armed services.

Useful links

The British Medical Association (BMA).
www.bma.org.uk

The careers service of the British Medical Journal
www.bmjcareers.com

The home NHS homepage for Modernising Medical Careers
www.mmc.nhs.uk

The Conference of Postgraduate Medical Deans (COPMeD)
www.copmed.org.uk

The Postgraduate Medical Education and Training Board
www.pmetb.org.uk

The General Medical Council
www.gmc-uk.org

Medical careers in the armed services:

Royal Navy
www.royal-navy.mod.uk/static/pages/3355.html

Army
www.army.mod.uk/careers/officer/jd_medical_officer.html

Royal Air Force
www.rafcareers.com/jobs/job_files/jobfile_medicalofficer.cfm

The financial implications of studying medicine: money matters

I've done a degree before, you are thinking, I know what kind of money it takes to go to University. But have your standards of living moved on since then? Are baked beans on toast not so familiar anymore? Medicine is notoriously the most costly course to undertake at university, but graduate entry medical courses present an extra dimension of financial considerations. You may have recently completed your undergraduate degree, in which case your pre-existing student debts may still be hanging over you. Or you may have graduated years ago and have considerable earning power and savings with which to support yourself during this next degree. Either way, there is a standard gamut of costs you will need to manage, and equally a standard range of available funds. The financial assistance available to each graduate entry student differs vastly because a person's assets, income, age and personal circumstance (such as family, dependents and disability) all affect the amount of financial assistance you can get from the governmental coffers. Here we detail the kind of costs you will encounter and how you might pave a way through them while minimising a potential cash haemorrhage.

What you will need the money for
As a student, there is more to life than simple living costs, books and a bit of photocopying. The entire process of graduate entry medicine, from medical school applications to job applications, as well as trying to look the part of a wannabe doctor, all costs money. There are plenty of things that you may not have considered, such as stethoscopes, the cost of

undertaking an elective and travel for clinical placements.

Application and preparation costs.

The largest financial demands at this stage are the application fees for certain entrance exams, where applicable. There are also additional costs such as the UCAS application fee, postage and enquiries with individual universities, travel costs incurred on attending Open Days, and, if all goes well, interviews. Eight of the fourteen graduate entry courses have an associated entrance exam. The details of these are found in chapter 8, but in brief, at the time of writing, BMAT costs £21.50 for UK applicants and £46.00 for other candidates, GAMSAT costs £176 and MSAT costs £75. At present the UCAS application fee is £5 if you are applying to only one university for one course, or £15 if you are applying to more than one university. Cambridge has an additional £15 application fee and Oxford an additional £10 application fee. In preparing for entrance exams and interviews you may wish to buy some appropriate reading material, as detailed in chapters 8 and 9.

Once you gain a place to study medicine, the cash will have no difficulty finding places to be frittered away. The prices quoted in this chapter are correct for the 2006-2007 academic year.

Tuition fees

The 2006 academic year sees the introduction of increased tuition fees for courses commencing that year and thereafter. There will be a cap of £3,000 per year (for Home students; see below for further explanation), set for the whole of the next Parliament, so the maximum fee will not rise by more than the rate of inflation before 2010 at the earliest. Universities will be allowed to vary the fees to below £3000 should they wish, but at the time of writing all medical course tuition fees are set to £3000. Given the expense of medical training, this is unlikely to be reduced.

At present, graduate entry students, like all students, must pay their tuition fees up front. However, commencing in 2006 and in line with the increase in fees, the Government is introducing a tuition fees payment scheme of deferred payment upon graduation, with accumulated inflationary interest. Eligible students can apply for a Student Loan for Fees. The loans are to be repaid upon graduation when you will pay 9% of any income you earn above £15,000. Alternatively, you may opt to pay your tuition fees to the University directly, at the start of each year of study, either in full or through the University approved instalment scheme. There are to be no upper age limits imposed for this scheme. However, it is not yet clear whether graduate entry students who have already availed themselves of this scheme during their first undergraduate degree will still have access to the scheme during their second degree as a graduate entry medical student.

The tuition fee usually includes registration, tuition and examination. Such course fees are determined by the individual universities and the amount you have to pay is determined by your status as Home, EU or International student. Your status as a Home or International classification is decided by the universities to which you apply; it is essential that you check with the individual university to ascertain your status.

On the whole, most universities define a Home student as one who is domiciled in the UK. You would need to show that you have the right of abode or indefinite leave to enter or remain in the UK, or a passport stamp which gives you the right of readmission to the UK. You need to have been 'ordinarily resident' in the UK throughout the three years immediately before the start of your course and the reason for your residence during that period should not have been wholly for the purpose of receiving full-time education. At most universities, an EU national who has been resident in the European Economic Area (EEA) throughout the three year period, for reasons other than full-time education, would also be classed as a Home student.

Most other students who do not fall within the Home Student or EU classification would be considered as International Students and be liable to pay considerably higher fees. Some graduate entry medicine courses exclude International Student applicants. At the time of writing those schools *accepting* international applicants are King's College London, Oxford University, Queen Mary University of London, University of Southampton and University of Warwick. An international student could be asked to pay tuition fees anywhere between £10,000 - £25,000 per year, incrementally increasing with each ensuing year of the course.

If you are a UK Home student you should apply for a tuition fee loan through your Local Education Authority. The following website provides more information: www.dfes.gov.uk/studentsupport

If you are an EU student you should contact the Department for Education and Skills (DfES) EU team at EUTeam@dfes.gsi.gov.uk, or visit: www.dfes.gov.uk/studentsupport/eustudents

It is unfortunately very unclear how the proposed changes will affect existing financial assistance for graduate entry medical students - that is, whether the NHS bursary scheme (as detailed below) will change, particularly under the increasing demand of more graduate entry medical courses.

Living costs

We feel that it is beneath our readership to attempt to explain what living costs you ought to consider. Accommodation costs are detailed in the relevant University sections of chapter 3. The British Medical Association completed a survey in 2004 of medical student expenditure and found some enlightening facts that might assist in your own planning:

> *The average monthly accommodation cost outside London was £265, while inside London it was £351.*

> *The average medical student's day-to-day living expenditure was £360-570 per month*

Studying costs

The process of graduating from a medical degree demands different costs in each year or stage.

In year one you will mostly incur set-up costs. The materials you will need include a stethoscope (ranging in price from £30-150), at least one decent set of clothes (since most graduate entry courses send you to interact with patients in the first year), and what will seem like a small library of books. You will borrow and buy books throughout your degree but the biggest surge in book buying tends to be the basics in first year, then the clinical guides and finals revision materials in the penultimate and final year. How much do medical students really spend on books? Whether they be new or second hand, book costs can range from the low hundreds of pounds up to a thousand pounds. You will also need to set up your stationery supplies. Indeed, such things as lever arch files are going to start growing like an unwelcome fungus over your entire room. Although all Universities provide computing facilities, you may find you would prefer a home computer to work on.

When you reach the penultimate and final year of your course you will be spending the majority of your time in the clinical setting, so you will need to expand your wardrobe to include a few more smarts. Your travel costs to clinical placements will escalate and you may need to stay in on-site hospital accommodation or GP accommodation which you may have to pay for initially before possible reimbursement by your University.

At the end of the degree you will have to emerge through the flaming hoops of finals exams, hopefully with degree in hand. At the last hurdle, there are countless revision books you may be seduced to buy. The expense you are least likely to resist is the one that plays most on your fears: finals revision courses. For instance, The Medical Defence Union (MDU) and the Medical Protection Society (MPS) run courses all around the country to assist final year students in preparing for the finals exams. Many students find them irresistible. With a membership discount they can cost around £90-£250 per course.

Elective costs

One of the brightest blips on your radar as a medical student is the elective period. This is your chance to travel to fascinating far-flung places and experience life and medicine in a different context. Although some students choose to stay in the UK for their elective, the majority choose to go abroad. In general the elective period lasts between 3-12 weeks, but some courses offer no elective period - it all depends on your University. Although the cost of an elective will vary depending on your destination, you might expect a *minimum* expense to be well above the thousand pound mark.

During your elective period, travel, accommodation, living expenses, plus all the extra costs of being in a new and exciting place (such as health insurance, HIV prophylaxis of about £100 and visas), can run into thousands of pounds. Many universities offer financial assistance to students for elective, but these funds are not available to everyone and are not always that sizeable. You would be wise to assume that you will have to find your own funding for your elective. This could come from your own shallow pockets, or you could apply to external sources for assistance. Indeed, some of the Medical Societies mentioned later in this chapter give to students for their elective period. www.medicsworld.co.uk offers elective advice including a list of the various organizations offering financial awards for elective travel.

Clinical placement costs

The average non-London medical student spends £558 per year on travel between lectures, clinical attachments and home, while the London medical student spends £699 per year. The Department of Health provides funding to your medical school to assist in funding clinical placements. This includes a small portion of money for your travel and on-site accommodation costs. For details of the rates, see the *Financial help for health care students* document on the DoH website listed below.

Society memberships

Should you feel the need to network and broaden your horizons, medical societies such as the British Medical Association (BMA) can offer excellent sources of information and contact with the medical world which you will soon be entering. Other societies include the Royal Society of Medicine (RSM), and if you are female, the Medical Women's Federation (MWF). These societies charge between £20-30 per annum for student membership.

The BMA News would keep you abreast of how the medical profession operates and changes, and reading the letters page can give you an idea of the prevailing opinions of working doctors and students. Also, these societies offer money prizes to medical students with obvious financial and CV advantages to the winners. The RSM run teaching courses in a wide range of relevant medical areas including medical ethics, politics and careers, all of which certainly help broaden your approach to medicine.

Where the money will come from.
The two primary government sources of funding are the Department for Education and Skills (DfES) and the Department of Health (DoH).

The DfES website contains updated information on their standard available funds (detailed below):

- *Student Loan for Maintenance*
- *Student Loan for Fees*
- *Maintenance Grant*
- *The DfES website: www.dfes.gov.uk/studentsupport/students/200_2006_entry.shtml*

The DoH document *Financial help for health care students* (see www.dh.gov.uk) contains the specifications of their standard available fund, the NHS bursary (detailed below).

For students starting their course in September 2006 or later, the Government will write off student loan balances (except for arrears) which are left unpaid 25 years after their liability to repay commenced, which is the April after the course finished. This will cover both Student Loans for Fees as well as Student Loans for Maintenance.

All other funding comes from a wide range of sources detailed later in this section.

Department for Education and Skills
The DfES makes financial support available for students. In the new

scheme of Government support, which hopes to widen access to people from lower income families, the amount of help you can receive depends on household income. From 2006 onwards help will come in two forms:

1) Maintenance Grant
2) Student Loan for Maintenance

The amount you can access of each type of support depends on household income.

Table 1. Maintenance Grant amounts

Household income	Maintenance Grant
£17,500	£2,700
£26,500	£1,200
£37,500	Nil
£50,000	Nil

Table 2. 2006-2007 Student Loan for Maintenance amounts

	Student living at home	Student living away from home, in London	Student living away from home, outside London
Maximum full year student loan for maintenance	£3,415	£6,170	£4,405
Maximum *final* year student loan for maintenance	£3,085	£5,620	£4,080

The Maintenance Grant is exactly that; a non-repayable grant. It is expected that around half of all new full-time students are likely to be eligible for a full or partial Maintenance Grant, but the amount depends on your income and the income of your household.

The Student Loan is a loan administered by the Student Loans Company (SLC) which accrues interest at the rate of inflation, i.e. 2.6%, and will be repayable on graduation. Maintenance Grant recipients' entitlement to the student loan for maintenance will be reduced by up to £1,200 because up to £1,200 of the maintenance grant is paid in substitution for part of the maintenance loan (which has the effect of reducing the debt for lower income students by up to £1,200 a year). Students who receive the full Maintenance Grant and who are on courses charging the £3,000 fee (i.e. graduate entry medical courses) will get at least £300 a year additional financial support from their university or college in the form of a bursary, making a total package of non-repayable DfES support of at least £3,000 per year. Eligibility for these funds is assessed by the

Local Education Authority (LEA).
The household income will be measured against your status as 'dependent' or 'independent'. Dependent students are those whose parents' income is taken into account. Independent students are aged over 25, or have been married before the start of the academic year for which they are applying for support, or have supported themselves for at least three years, or have no living parents.

Additional sources of help from the DfES/LEA include:
- *Parent's Learning Allowance- up to £1,365*
- *Child Tax Credit- paid by Inland Revenue*
- *Adult Dependent's Grant- up to £2,395 for full-time students with adult dependents*
- *Childcare Grant- Up to £5967 for one child, or up to £8840 for two or more children.*

However, being in receipt of the NHS bursary (detailed below) does affect eligibility for a number of these allowances.

The Student Loan for Fees is detailed in the first section of this chapter.

Hardship and Access Funds
The DfES has made funding available from Access and Hardship Funds with priority to particular groups of students such as those with children, especially lone parents, students with disability, mature students and those in their final year etc.

Hardship Loans are paid in addition to a full student loan after recommendation from the University. They are administered by the Student Loans Company. Usually, the maximum amount available is £500 per year, but students are not required to apply for the full amount. Applications for Hardship Loans can usually only be made once a normal SLC loan has been received. The eligibility requirements are the same as for the SLC loan but you need to demonstrate to your university that you are in real financial difficulty and need help. Hardship loans are added to your account with the SLC and repaid in the same way as the main student loan. They are often restricted to Home/EU students.

In addition to the Hardship Loan you can receive a Hardship Fund. The DfES has given universities money to provide selective help, at the University's discretion, to students who have serious financial problems.

Access bursaries are intended to provide additional financial help to students with dependent children. Non-repayable bursaries of up to £500 may be granted to students who are awarded a Dependents Allowance for a child by their LEA. The primary purpose of the bursaries is to help with childcare costs but they can be used to help with other course-related expenses such as travel and books.

Department of Health/NHS bursary

The single, largest source of available funding for many students of graduate entry medicine is the NHS bursary provided by the Department of Health. The bursary provides for maintenance costs and, at the time of writing, tuition fees. Eligibility criteria are detailed in the DoH document, but on the whole it is for home students or students who have been resident in *England* for 3 years prior to commencement of the course. Whether the bursary will continue to cover tuition fees during the new 2006 implementation is not presently declared by the DoH. The current DoH document states that it will contribute £1,150 towards tuition fees, but it does not state whether it will increase that amount to £3,000 in 2006.

The bursary is means tested. For students aged under 25 at the start of the academic year it is assessed against parental income, whereas for independent students, parental income is not assessed but a spouse's contribution may be. The DoH bursary can be taken in years 2-4 of the graduate entry programme. These bursaries restrict the amount of student loan (LEA/SLC loan) that will be made available to you while in receipt of the bursary. If you are an EU national you may not normally qualify for a bursary. You may not be eligible to receive the DoH/NHS bursary if you take an intercalated BSc year during your graduate entry programme.

Although the DoH publishes a guide to the amount you can expect, it is difficult to determine the breakdown. The means-tested maintenance amount, i.e. the basic bursary, for London students per annum is £2,837 and for non-London students is £2,309p.a. This amount is increased with the following extra additions to the basic bursary:

- *an additional amount per week of course above 30 weeks duration; £96p.w. for London students, £74p.w. for non-London students*
- *Older Student's Allowance (£406 aged 26, £704 aged 27, £1045 aged 28 and £1,381 aged 29 and over)*
- *Dependent's Allowance: £2,393p.a. for a dependent spouse and up to £1,915p.a. for dependent children*
- *Single Students with Dependants: £1,181p.a.*
- *Childcare Allowance: pays childcare for up to £170p.w. for two or more children.*
- *Disabled Student's Allowance: up to £11,838p.a. for a helper and extra for equipment and travel*
- *Clinical Placement Costs: reimbursement for car, motorbike, bicycle usage to travel to clinical placements*

Funding for overseas graduate entry students is limited.

Scholarships

Individual universities have their own scholarships, such as Vice-Chancellor's Scholarships for excellence in sport and music. They will also have scholarships unique to that institution, the details of which can be gathered from the respective University. One to look out for is the alumni scholarship, especially if the University at which you are studying graduate entry medicine is your alma mater!

Charitable foundations

It is a little known fact that there is a considerable source of available funds held in charitable organizations that could be accessed by most students of graduate entry medicine. However, as relatively few students know of the various charitable organizations and even fewer students can be bothered to trawl through the application process, much of this potential funding goes untapped. Some of the information below is sourced from The Education Grants Advisory Service (EGAS) whose website is denoted later in the chapter.

There are numerous charities and trusts that provide bursaries, scholarships, fellowships and funds to students. The criteria for eligibility set by trusts are extremely diverse. Most trusts make relatively small awards, while a very few trusts are prepared to sponsor students throughout the duration of a course. Many trusts have a limited remit such as only assisting study leading to a particular profession, study at a specific academic level, those living in or originating from a specific geographical area, falling within a specific age range or those of a specified religion. Trusts can seldom help with an immediate financial crisis.

The procedure for applying to trusts differs widely although most trusts require either a letter or application form. If there is no clear guidance given by the trust, you should write to the trust detailing the type of funding required, your personal circumstances and academic background, including relevant supporting evidence. Before applying to a trust always check eligibility criteria. The vast majority of trusts require an applicant to meet 'qualifying' criteria which might be specific to one or more of the following: age, sex, religion, subject of study, country of birth, parents' occupation, etc. Do not waste your own and the trust's time by submitting an application for which you are not truly eligible. Keep in mind that you usually need a confirmed place at University before your application will be considered. Do not apply to every charity in the same year because the charities know each other and tend only to offer money to those not in receipt of moneys from any other source.

If you are fortunate to receive an award from the trusts, write and thank them, and list it on your CV. And since more people apply every year, the charities need further funding each year. Once you graduate, have paid off your loans and are just about to retire, you could make your own contribution back to the fund that helped you get through medical studies in the first place!

There are too many charities and trusts to list in this book, but some of the better known charities that support graduate entry medical students include The Sir Richard Stapeley Educational Trust (their remit is to support graduate entry students), The Sidney Perry Foundation (they only support students on a second degree), The Foulkes Foundation (for medical students who completed a PhD prior to becoming a medical student), The Professional Classes Aid Council (they support during the clinical years only) and The Society for Promoting Training of Women (they support women in the clinical years). Many of these charities offer £300 - £3,000 p.a.

The best list of charities and trusts can be found via The Education Grants Advisory Services (EGAS) of the Family Welfare Association which gives information and advice on potential sources of educational funding. The EGAS was established in 1962 to offer students, especially disadvantaged students, expert guidance and advice to enable them to secure funding for education and training. Their website has an excellent search engine, which sifts through 956 Trusts then finds relevant Trusts for you to contact based on your own personal information and circumstances.

Website: www.egas-online.org/fwa/
Contact: EGAS
Grants Department
Family Welfare Association
501-505 Kingsland Road
London E8 4AU
Tel: 0207 254 6251

Potential funding for elective

The Royal Colleges and other professional associations offer monetary awards to medical students who may have an interest in that specialty. The Colleges won't give you money for nothing: you will have to work for it! They usually reward the winning entry of an essay competition with £100 - £800. All of these colleges and countless other sources of funding for a medical elective are listed on the BMA's 'Directory of sources for funding an elective':

www.bma.org.uk/ap.nsf/Content/Medicalelectivescontactinfo.

Some of the better known charities that support medical student electives include The Roger & Sarah Bancroft Clark Charitable Trust and The Vandervell Foundation.

Commercial bank loans

High street banks offer professional studies loans, usually from the second year of the course onwards, but only 30% of medical students have a commercial bank loan on graduating. However, those that do average a graduating loan of £7,660. High street banks also tend to have loans specifically for elective costs. With a professional studies loan, repayments would commonly commence 6months - 1 year after graduation, with interest charged somewhere near but above the bank's base rate.

A career development loan is also a deferred repayment high street bank loan, but while you are studying the Department for Education and Skills (DfES) pays the interest. For further information go to the website on Career Development Loans at www.lifelonglearning.co.uk/cdl. You will also find there an excellent student life budget planner, which reminds you of otherwise forgettable costs. Most students wait until they are in the desperate final stages of their last year of medical studies to take out a commercial loan. As a student you also benefit from the option of having a student bank account which confers larger than usual overdraft options. Given that 65% of medical students have an overdraft on graduating, this may prove a worthwhile facility. The average medical student overdraft on graduating is £1,462.

Work part-time

Shocking though it might seem to some, working part-time whilst studying for an intensive graduate entry medical degree is actually achievable. It will require considerable time management skills, but balancing part-time work with full-time classes can be rewarding both financially and professionally. It can be particularly beneficial if you find part-time work in medicine, or allied to it. For example, you might find work at your hospital as a Medical Secretary/Administrator or as an Auxiliary Nurse. This can improve your breadth of medical knowledge and keep you up to speed on the ward environment. You can be reassured by the knowledge that 61% of medical students work part-time or during their holidays (BMA 2004 survey data).

Student discounts

If being an undergraduate student is a hazy memory for you, you may have forgotten about student discount cards. This is one of the perks of student life! Your National Union of Students (NUS) card will gain you discounts of about 10% on products from many companies. You can find more information at the NUS website: www.nusonline.co.uk. Do not forget that as a full-time student you can also get student discounts on rail travel (using a Young Person's Railcard) and other transport services. You will also have access to student discounted travel through the STA travel company, which is handy in minimizing the costs of your elective. There are numerous hidden student discounts that are easily unearthed with a little bit of effort. For example, if you live in a house with only students you will be exempt from paying council tax.

The overall picture

Sobering facts have recently been produced by the British Medical Association from its survey of medical student finances. For students commencing in 2006 with the new tuitions fees, it is estimated that upon graduation medical students may accrue up to £28,000 of debt including payment of their own £3000 annual tuition fees. Admittedly these estimates are for standard course students who receive less NHS bursary, but they in part reflect the increasing cost of medical education.

The hard facts set out in this chapter may be enough to put some people off the financial risks and investment that are required to study medicine as a graduate. But choosing to study medicine is not a financial decision; it is born of far deeper passions. A career in medicine is sheltered by relative stability and security. Some might find it encouraging to now turn to the NHS pay scales for doctors that are set out in chapter 4; you will one day be able to pay off all the costs mentioned here!

Relevant Work Experience

Work experience should be very much about quality and not quantity. Equally, the quality does not relate to the seniority or prestige of your responsible superior or mentor, but to what you actually do and what you learn from it. The gold standard is to spend time as a care assistant in a nursing home or similar, so that you get the chance to spend time with sick people who may be frustrated and confused; exactly what you will have to deal with as a junior doctor. In addition, it is sterling to have witnessed a good doctor in action. Do you have some the same skills as that doctor? Are you frustrated by a patient who is 'causing' their own illness or impassioned by the knowledge that they are someone's beloved mother and as much in need and as valuable as the next person? You will have thoughts on these issues already, but they will become far more profound when framed in the context of hands-on work experience. Candidates might find it useful to keep a diary of their experiences, not so much in terms of a list of where they were and when, but of feelings associated with specific patients and experiences, and this can be useful to freshen your feelings and reactions prior to interview.

Why Work Experience?

As mentioned in chapter 2, the reason for obtaining relevant work experience is not simply to satisfy the medical schools' requirements, but to be as certain as you possibly can be that medicine is the right choice for you. Embarking on a medical career, especially as a mature individual, is an enormous commitment, and you would not be the first graduate entry student to feel that they have used up their life's quota of mistakes and wanderings. Most candidates reading this book cannot afford, either emotionally or financially, to make a poor decision with something so hugely important.

It is true that without work experience you are extremely unlikely to be able to write a convincing personal statement, or compete at interview. Yet it is curious how many candidates are convinced of their desire to be a doctor, when their knowledge of the subject barely extends beyond their personal experiences of having their appendix removed and of nursing their grandfather for a few days after his hip replacement.

Conversely, do not think that you are necessarily in a better position simply because you are able to produce a long list of different experiences with different eminent Consultants. Whilst variety is great, the benefit of work experience comes from a far more humble insight than a seemingly showy list of contacts.

What experiences are you seeking?
This is the question most candidates ask, but it is the wrong one. The question you should be asking yourself is 'what should I be learning from my experiences?' You may think that the ex-NHS bed manager or paramedic necessarily has better experiences. Whilst it's true to say that these experiences are certainly the Black and Decker power drill of possible experiences, it doesn't mean that they're any better at hanging the door than you are with your humble screw driver.

Satisfactory demonstration of attributes such as empathy, intellectual ability, willingness to accept responsibility, ability to handle stress, communication, teamwork and so on is not dependent on the type of experience, but of your analysis, criticism and insight into a given experience. This is true for any question that requires you to draw upon your experiences. Experience in a medical environment is of course preferable. But you can use other things if need be. If you've worked well in a team, or had to communicate difficult information and so on, then be proud of it as a positive reflection of transferable skills relevant to medicine.

During your chosen experiences, you should try to seize the opportunity to gain an understanding in as many aspects of healthcare as you can. This may include:

- *Being able to recognise and empathise with many of the needs of patients*
- *Communicate with patients and the medical staff, where appropriate*
- *Recognise what makes a good doctor*
- *Recognise the skills that you have that reflect those of a good doctor*
- *Make the most of any opportunities to develop those skills*
- *Recognise the importance of the multi-disciplinary team*
- *Consider the problems facing patients, relatives, doctors and other healthcare professionals*
- *Consider your own prejudices, fears and concerns (everyone has them)*

This is by no means an exhaustive list of issues that you might dwell on during your work experience. Indeed, a list somewhat detracts from the preferred notion that you gain an understanding that is an intricately woven ensemble of practicalities, emotions, finances, ethics and management issues.

Useful sources of work experience

There are many opportunities through which you will be able to gain real insight into some of the issues listed above.

Care Work

- *Care work/ care assistant at residential home/ care home for the elderly/disabled (e.g. residential care home for children with autism)*
- *Volunteer at hospital/ volunteer auxiliary/ ward volunteer*

- *Volunteer at a soup kitchen, centre for the homeless*
- *Mentoring and tutoring*
- *Volunteer Counselling*
- *Befriending services to disadvantaged/ elderly*
- *Community work*

These are simply some ideas to hopefully spark your own imagination, or nudge you in a useful direction. There is no suggestion that you do all of these things. For some more thoughtful people, just one type of high quality experience may be sufficient for them to gain the sort of insight that is encouraged. However, even this type of candidate is likely to need to spend a significant period of time in their role. Indeed, Bristol University actually state that candidates should consider at least 3 months' experience as a Healthcare Assistant or similar.

Shadowing

Although shadowing rarely affords any hands-on exposure, there is no doubt that shadowing a doctor will clearly give you insight into their work. It cannot replace care work or similar, but provides a valuable adjunct opportunity. You could also learn a great deal from shadowing other healthcare professionals. For instance, if you gain shadowing experience at your local General Practice, try to observe the Community Nurses, in addition to the GP. Similarly, you may find that working with physiotherapists could be a rewarding opportunity, and so forth. Many candidates get very excited about the prospect of spending time with, say, a top Consultant Neurosurgeon. Of course, you would not turn down this opportunity, as it is a wonderful one, but bare in mind the limitations of what it tells you about an average patient's needs and an average doctor's workload. Also, those doctors who are now consultants were medical students when trends were different, and they may inadvertently encourage an 'unfashionable' outlook. You may find it more relevant to attempt to spend time with a more recently qualified doctor and to spend time 'on take' (i.e. responsible for all hospital admissions during that shift). You could always go for the trial by fire approach and spend a Friday night shift in A&E.

Other useful experiences and opportunities through work and current hobbies.
You may be able to additionally demonstrate some skills by other means, for instance fundraising for charity or gaining a first aid at work certificate. These types of experiences can often be undertaken through work, and is thus particularly useful for the busy professional and/or parent/spouse. Similarly, for those candidates who play sport, you may find that there are some very rewarding opportunities if you simply change the emphasis of your training. For instance, try performing an internet search on your own sport, with other keywords such as disability, children and volunteer. There are huge opportunities for you to be involved in worthwhile work, which should be rewarding irrespective of you ultimate aim.

Experiences for candidates already working in a healthcare setting
If you are currently a pharmacist, PhD student, NHS manager, social worker or any other professional involved with patients, healthcare or research, you will clearly have extensive insight into your particular field. However, your role could be narrow, and also biased. Particularly for those working in a relatively closeted research environment, gaining hands-on care experience is important. Aside from improving your insight, you will be able to more easily demonstrate yourself to be a well-rounded, interested and motivated individual with demonstrable human qualities.

Reading
Although not strictly work experience, it is useful to include here the notion of reading widely. In much the same way as your medical knowledge develops at medical school, your understanding of current

affairs and advancements in medicine will be superior if built over time. Read relevant newspaper articles, perhaps subscribe to a journal, and maintain objectivity by always considering the different impacts on all parties affected by any article that you read. Indeed, when reading a newspaper article on a recent development consider what it means to patients. You might then read more detailed information on the subject (an old but classic example would be to explore the MMR vaccine debate by reading Andrew Wakefield's original paper in the Lancet journal then read the responses which followed in the media). The General Medical Council (GMC) and British Medical Association (BMA) websites provide an enormous wealth of fascinating material relating to the provision of healthcare.

Personal Experiences

Although not work experience as such, your insight into medicine through your own personal experience as a relative or carer may be very useful. If these experiences form a large part of your desire to become a doctor, it may be worth taking the time to think about your unique situation from other people's point of view and to try, in so far as it's possible, to put the experience into more objective and general terms. Taking time to reflect and articulate on these experiences prior to interview can be very useful.

How to obtain work experience

Care Experience

You need to obtain this work experience as soon as possible. For one reason, this type of experience is not like cramming for an exam; you need to absorb the experiences over time. Also, you are likely to have to undergo a formal application procedure which will include an extensive and time consuming police check, as well as possible application forms, interviews and basic training.

In order to find a suitable 'host', you might start by performing an internet search using relevant key words such as 'care assistant', 'volunteer', 'nursing', 'disabled' and so forth. It can then often be most efficient to telephone an organisation in the first instance, such that you can target your application, become known to the relevant department, or be alerted to the fact that the organisation is unsuitable. There are numerous agencies you could contact who deploy carers in the healthcare setting.

Do highlight the fact that you are volunteering (if that is what you are doing). Most institutions do not have extensive funds and extra help can be gratefully received. However, there is significant administrative hassle for the institution just to accept a volunteer so you may find that you have to prove yourself more than you expected. Nevertheless, this is a good opportunity to practise demonstrating your interest and commitment to healthcare.

Shadowing

If shadowing, you are less likely to need to undergo police checks and formal application procedures than as a care worker, so invariably shadowing experience can be obtained relatively quickly. If you have any contacts with medics, they may be willing to help you. Your own GP may be willing to pass you to a colleague in another surgery (they are unlikely to allow you to shadow within your home practice due to obvious confidentiality issues).

In order to shadow doctors in hospital, you might approach a number of hospitals. You will find some very helpful and others less so. If you telephone and ask to speak to someone who deals with work experience or voluntary services you may find someone helpful. Also, most hospitals have a good Patient Advice and Liaison Service (PALS). They offer patient advice and support, and deal with comments and complaints. They are often enthusiastic about your interest, will provide valuable information and help you to find other useful contacts.

Some hospitals are so inundated with requests for work experience that they provide specific programmes. These are often designed with school leavers in mind and are therefore often organised for the start of the summer. However, if you are too late, you might at least be able to speak to the organiser who will clearly have good insight into your needs.

Candidates (well, those nearing the application deadline without relevant experience) invariably moan about how difficult it is to get work experience. It isn't. It just takes a bit of time and perseverance, motivation and a positive outlook.

How to get the most from your work experience
If you refer to chapter 2 you will start to gain insight into what makes a good doctor, and the reality of studying medicine. Chapter 7 and 9 highlight what the medical schools are looking for and how you might demonstrate those qualities. If you read *Tomorrow's Doctors* alongside the medical school prospectuses, you will gain an even more detailed view of what makes a good doctor.

For all of the skills mentioned throughout this book and elsewhere, try to witness and achieve them during your work experience. Empathise with patients. Talk to them, listen to their needs. Ask them about their care. Be kind. Be thoughtful. Be responsible. Talk to other healthcare professionals. Empathise with them too. What are the problems facing doctors, other healthcare professionals, patients and their relatives? How do you feel about financial constraints? How do you feel about the patient who is largely 'responsible' for their own illness? Do you think they are owed a lesser standard of care or are they an equal individual? How do you feel about sickness, suffering and death? How do you feel about bodily fluids, unsightly conditions and nasty smells?

You may find it very useful to keep a diary of your experiences. Whilst it might help you to note meetings and departments attended and so forth, the key use of your retrospective diary should be to note memorable moments and interesting patients, your own emotions, and things you have witnessed. When you write your personal statement, or prepare for interview, this collection of ideas and emotions will be of enormous help to you in relating your thoughts in a fresh and dynamic way.

For each of the examples and situations that you note in your diary, also try to empathise and rationalise the situation. Did the aggressive patient behave that way because he is a mean character or is there more to it than that? Was the doctor unkind? Were the patient and/or doctor frightened? Was the patient confused? Were they lonely? Were they on medication that might alter their mood? You may find that by communicating and empathising with that patient, you may not only answer these questions, you might also provide a great deal of support to a patient in need when other healthcare professionals simply cannot afford the time. Also try to think realistically about how you would feel if you were caring for such a patient in addition to many others.

Similarly, when you see a good doctor in action, think about every facet of why that doctor was good. What was their body language like? What questions did they ask? Did they listen and really pick up on the patient's underlying message? What information did they give? How did they give it? Why not ask patients what they think makes a good doctor? And most importantly, ask yourself if you have these qualities? Can you demonstrate them? Can you improve on them?

Be careful not to be a maverick and focus on the flaws of the system (for you will see many). Of course it can be easier and sometimes more natural to exemplify skills by considering the consequences of their absence. It is important to recognise inadequacies; they exist and one needs to be realistic. However, remember that, on balance, you should *want* to work within the NHS with patients and health care professionals, rather than feel that it is something you could simply *cope* with.

The Personal Statement

Part of the process of applying to university or college involves the submission of a 'personal statement' to the Universities & Colleges Admissions Service (UCAS; their website is www.ucas.co.uk). Most medical schools include consideration of your personal statement in their decision-making process. Even if your chosen schools will not read your personal statement, you should still think of the entire UCAS form as an opportunity to rationalise your desire to study medicine and as a chance to make a first impression. Writing a personal statement is seen by many as one of the most difficult parts of the UCAS form.

Graduate entry medical schools using the UCAS Personal Statement (or personal statements on other supplementary forms) as part of their shortlisting process.

Birmingham	*Yes*
Bristol	*Yes*
Cambridge	*Yes*
Kings	*No*
Leicester	*Yes*
Liverpool	*Yes*
Newcastle	*Yes*
Nottingham	*No*
Oxford	*No*
Queen Mary	*Yes*
Southampton	*Yes*
St George's	*No*
Swansea	*Yes*

Warwick   *Yes*

NB. King's will read your personal statement for consideration for the standard entry course.

What sorts of things should go into your Personal Statement?
Some people fear that they will never have enough material, whilst others feel that the space is far too small to allow himself or herself justice. Of course, some candidates just see how it works out. Whichever group you belong to, you will need to spend a significant amount of time on the statement and you should expect to revise your text many times before settling on the final form and content.

There is a lot of guidance available in the school prospectuses and websites about what qualities the medical school are looking for. Chapter 2 discusses in some detail the essence of *Tomorrow's Doctors*. Although different schools might place a slightly different emphasis on different skills, they are all seeking essentially the same common endpoint. That is not to say that all schools are looking for one type of person, but they *are* looking for candidates who demonstrate suitable potential. The qualities and characteristics likely to be of interest to a medical school, especially of a graduate applicant, might include:

- *Convincing explanation of the candidate's desire to study medicine*
- *Commitment to a career in medicine*
- *Intellectual and academic strength*
- *An empathic attitude*
- *Achievements (in addition to academic achievements)*
- *A realistic attitude about the profession and the course*
- *Self-motivation*
- *Evidence of an ability to apply oneself to a task*
- *Good organisational skills*

- *Growth as a person*
- *A 'well rounded' personality*
- *Demonstration of a wide range of interests*
- *Awareness of current developments*

These types of skills are all potential elements of a good personal statement; you should be able to make additions to this list after studying the medical school prospectuses and the first section of this book. A strong candidate will be able to demonstrate, largely from their work experience, why they would make a good doctor. Chapter 6 discusses how you might obtain good work experience.

Getting Started

Before actually beginning to draft your personal statement, or indeed before reading much more of this chapter, you may find it useful to carry a notebook with you and to start making a list of things about yourself that *might* form elements of your personal statement. Keep your list easily to hand and add to it whenever you have another idea concerning accomplishments, skills, abilities and things that you enjoy or excel at. The key at this point is to be completely uncritical about the contents of your list and to work on it over a period of time. Even if you start off with a sense of inadequacy in the face of this task, you will soon surprise yourself with what a unique and gifted person you turn out to be.

An extract from your list might end up looking something like this:

- *Voluntary work at a local hospice*
- *Research experience*
- *University hockey team*
- *Post-graduate degree*
- *6 months teaching in India*
- *Counselling certificate/Uni NightOwls counselling team*

- *Bronze DofE Year 10*
- *Etc*

Hopefully your list will be substantial if disorganised. Even an apparently trivial item may subsequently become useful.

While you are busy with this in your spare time, carry on reading this chapter. In a few days time, you will want to start converting your list into your personal statement.

What to Include
Even for the few schools who will not read your UCAS statement, your interviewers are likely to explore at least some if not all of the qualities that you should seek to include in your statement. Writing the statement may be your earliest chance to consider answers to fundamental questions. For this reason you will find some overlap between materials in this chapter and chapter 9 where interviews are discussed.

Why Medicine?
Some people find it easier to rephrase this question to 'When and how did you first become interested in medicine as a career?' It may be that you or someone important to you was very ill at some time in your past and the resultant experience of hospitals and doctors inspired you, perhaps you are already a healthcare professional wanting to advance your career, perhaps there was no defining moment, you just always wanted to do it. Whatever the case, you need to spend some time thinking about this aspect of your application. Avoid excuses for not having taken medicine as a school leaver, do not talk about what deterred you in the past, but explain what motivates you now.

Demonstrating Commitment

Although shadowing and wider reading each demonstrate a degree of commitment, the role of work experience cannot be overestimated. This topic is mentioned elsewhere in this book but it is such an important part of your personal statement that it is dealt with here as well. If you do not explain *'Why Medicine?'* your application will probably still receive serious consideration. If you have no relevant work experience to talk about, it is unlikely that any schools will consider you further so in many respects the paragraphs on this topic are the most important of your statement.

The worst case is that you are reading this with either insignificant or non-existent work experience. You must organise something as a matter of urgency, not least because you are otherwise considering making one of the most important decisions of your life on less than adequate information. You must not lie on your application, do not pretend to have experience that you do not have and do not take the risk of writing about work experience that you have not yet organised as if it is something you have actually done, no matter how tempting. *will* have to talk about this at interview and the interview panel is expert at spotting fabrications they have heard it all before.

If you are or have ever worked as a healthcare professional, avoid detailed lists of your responsibilities - the reader will already know these - a very brief outline is all that is necessary. Focus instead on the personal qualities you have developed and used in this role. It will strengthen your statement further if you can provide evidence that you have expanded your experience in a different department or context from your usual responsibilities.

Ideally you will have a range of different experiences of working with people in a caring environment. In your final version you may not have room to provide more than a fairly bald list, but in your earliest drafts of your personal statement include things such as

- *any specific responsibilities you had/have,*
- *what you learned (especially about yourself),*
- *how you feel about what you did,*
- *what was difficult,*
- *what you found especially rewarding and so on.*

Keep these longer drafts as they will be useful if you are called to interview.

Demonstrating organisation skills and application

If you have outstanding academic results from both school and university but no extramural activities to describe, you have a problem. Think about times in your life when you were already heavily loaded with work and responsibilities (whether academically, professionally or personally) but undertook other activities as well. A job in the evenings or at weekends to finance your degree, for example, or active membership of a club which involved regular meetings and occupied time, would be good examples

Are you a 'well-rounded' person?

This overlaps, but is still distinct from, the question above about organisational skills. Because of the stressful nature of the training and career you are applying for, medical schools want you to have an outlet in the form of leisure activities. Think about how you spend your leisure time and how you can present this well in your personal statement. This should be an activity that is separate from voluntary work, required activities and so on; something that is purely for you - maybe you enjoy running or playing in a jazz band, for example. Note also that any extracurricular activity which is/was not obviously detrimental to your academic achievement or professional success will demonstrate that you are able to organise your workload efficiently and effectively.

Ideally, you should be able to give both physical and intellectual leisure activities but do not worry if your activities tend towards one or the other. Essentially, you should be doing something other than watching TV or going to the pub with your friends ('socialising') with at least some of your free time.

Demonstrating altruism?

This may well be demonstrated by your voluntary work, for example. It is altruistic to give up your free time to helping others for no reward (except that of being able to mention it on your UCAS form, of course!). One successful candidate described going swimming each week with a paraplegic friend who was only allowed in the pool if she had an able-bodied companion. Hopefully, you have something to offer in this respect.

Drafting Your Personal Statement

Look back at the list that you have made in your notebook and work experience diary. You will want to discard some things immediately. As much as possible, use recent or current examples of activities. Organise the remaining items under broad headings. Exactly what these are will depend on your list but will certainly include 'Work Experience', 'Leisure Activities' and so on. Once you have done this you are ready to start drafting your personal statement. Try to produce one or two paragraphs for each heading. Do not worry about length at this point unless you find that you have little to say.

If your list is still worryingly short, now is the time to get friends to help out. You will get a better and more constructive response from almost everyone you ask if, instead of telling them that you want a list of things for your UCAS form, you ask 'What qualities do I have that make me unique?' Hopefully what they have to say about you will give you a few more ideas for yourself.

Dealing with negative content

Everyone will have weaknesses and gaps in their application. As a generalisation you should avoid highlighting these - if they matter that much, the schools to which you are applying will identify them anyway and you are wasting valuable words.

A common concern amongst graduate applicants is that of dismal A-level results. Medicine is an academically demanding course and A-level grades for school leavers are set correspondingly high. Poor performance in A-levels may well be the reason why you did not study medicine as your first degree. You must highlight your academic achievement since then. Remember that graduate entry courses are in part designed to widen access and many schools have already made the decision to ignore A-level results.

If you are still at university and so have no qualifications more recent than your A-levels, you should probably mention academic ability in some way. First and foremost, do not bother with excuses. Whatever the reason for your lack of effort, you got poor A-level results because you did not do the necessary work. Accept this brutal fact and move on. Your strength lies in the fact that you have changed the way you work as a result of your poor showing at A-level. You could say something like, 'studying at degree level has taught me how to organise my work load efficiently and to apply myself effectively to my work.' Acknowledgement of your inadequate A-levels is implied rather than explicit but, more importantly, you have shown yourself as someone who can modify their approach to a key area of their life.

If you have a weakness that you really feel you cannot avoid mentioning, try to treat it in a similar way and turn it into a strength.

The Style of your Statement

If you are lucky, your personal statement will be the first one the Admissions Tutor reads after coffee on Monday morning. If you are not, yours will be the last one he reads before tea on Friday afternoon. What makes your personal statement eye catching enough to be worth a closer look and maybe even an offer of an interview?

For example, 'At Primary school I was an elf in the Woodcraft Folk and particularly enjoyed camping and bivouacking' will certainly catch the eye of anyone reading your personal statement, but probably will not have quite the impact you were hoping for. It also begs the question; if you enjoyed it that much why do you not have a more recent example of the outdoor life to describe?

Alternatively, 'to fund my studies, I work as a juggler and fire-eater in a circus, in the evening shows, in the matinee performances at the weekend and full time during my vacations' (if true, of course), is not only eye-catching in itself as a fairly unusual skill and experience but also implies that you are working during term time and hence adds evidence for an ability to organise your work load efficiently.

Some people pick a slightly unconventional style of presentation for their statement as a means of capturing attention. Included later is an example of this sort of approach. This technique can work well but needs to be used with caution. Remember, your personal statement makes your first impression for you; be aware of this aspect of your statement when revising it.

The UCAS publication, *How to Apply* includes the information for mature students that 'you can ignore the columns in Sections 7A and 7B and use them as free space if you want.' This is an acknowledgment that mature students will have experiences that are valid and valuable but which do not fit easily into the format provided. For medicine, which is very oversubscribed, it may be more appropriate to stick to a conventional approach to the space available to you as it makes the information more immediately accessible to the Admissions Tutor.

Similarly, although some sources of advice suggest that bullet points might be a useful approach to the restricted space of the personal statement, this approach may not be appropriate here. Firstly, bullet points are neither easier to read nor less demanding of space than a piece of continuous prose. Secondly, one of the skills that medical schools are interested in is your communication skills. A straightforward piece of writing with a restricted word count on a specified subject is an excellent test of basic communications skills. Make sure you pass this one with flying colours.

Revising your first draft

Go back to the websites and prospectuses for your chosen schools and find a list of things they are looking for in applicants. Compare this list to your personal statement - have you included everything they are looking for? If not, go back to your initial list, did you leave something helpful out? Add in the necessary material to your draft to satisfy all specified requirements.

Read over your text looking for any repetition of information that is found elsewhere on the form and remove it. The sole exception to this should be relevant work experience.

Get a red pen or a highlighter pen and mark every occurrence of the word 'I' and look for alternative ways of beginning sentences to get rid of all but one or two beginning 'I'. Then look for alternative vocabulary for words you have repeated noticeably.

Further Revisions

The second version may be longer than your first if you have added in more material to satisfy specifics for one or more institutions. Read through carefully and start to get a feel for whether or not you have placed the emphasis correctly. Listing modules from your degree, for example, is of minimal value and interest; that one sentence you put in about spending last summer working for Riding for the Disabled says far more of importance about you and deserves expansion.

If you are content that the emphasis and balance of the various elements is about right, start to think about word count. You should be aiming for around 500 words for your statement to fill the space provided neatly but without looking too crowded. You will probably find that the statement is far too long so you need to get really ruthless at this point.

Look for material that you can omit without leaving a significant gap in your presentation. Look for rambling and unfocused sentences and tighten up your use of language. Generally, try to use strong, positive sentences. Keep reducing the content until the word count is approximately correct ($\pm$50 words).

The Opening Statement

Do you have a strong opening sentence or paragraph? Now is the time to really think about this. If you can get this right you will make an immediate, positive impact on your reader. Some successful, graduate entry applicants have agreed that we can quote from their personal statements. Here are the opening 100 - 200 words from a selection of these. Look at each of these statements critically. What makes them strong? What weakens them in your opinion?

Example 1:

I am a practising State Registered Paramedic, currently employed by the Tees, East and North Yorkshire Ambulance Service NHS Trust. Prior to this I have worked in similar roles for other NHS ambulance services.

I am now reaching the limit of clinical development available to me within my current profession but I wish to continue to advance and mature as a practitioner and a healthcare professional. It is important to me that I can continue to work with people and I feel that I can best realise my own potential and also maximise the level of care that I am able to offer to patients by retraining as a doctor.

This is very good. A strong opening consisting of a clear but brief description of the author's current role and then a good rationale for retraining to be a doctor.

Example 2:

After working in management consultancy for five years, I have decided that I want to pursue a career in a caring profession. The primary reason is that, whilst I have enjoyed my job and been successful, I have found my voluntary activities in caring roles to be far more fulfilling. I have worked university holidays as a nurse in elderly and psychiatric wards, volunteered for a year at a weekend session for mentally ill individuals, and have spent the last 9 months volunteering at a London hospital on the elderly and now the admissions ward.

This is a weak opening statement - the author's job and years of employment are elsewhere on the form. They would get a better starting point if they began 'Whilst I have enjoyed my job . . . etc'. University holidays were at least 5 year ago. Although very useful and relevant, they should have focused attention onto the more recent experiences and given the old stuff a much less prominent position.

Example 3:

Having a physiology degree and full time employment experience within a hospital environment I have decided to pursue a career in medicine. I feel that my academic and work experience has given me a true idea about the realities of studying for and pursuing a career in medicine, which may not have been apparent at a younger age.

I gained a II.i in my physiology degree, modules included; metabolic, renal, exercise, CNS and reproductive physiology. My dissertation consisted of a literature review regarding the physiological mechanisms of pain relief and a research project evaluating the effect of age on left ventricular hypertrophy. In September 2004 I qualified as a Donor Care Physiologist at Papworth Hospital, Cambridge.

Rather weak. Much of the statement consisted of detailed lists similar to the ones shown above. Most of the material was irrelevant to their application and the important and relevant information buried under a mass of detail.

Example 4:

This is something that I have always wanted to do since I was a child, and if it were not for a change of rules that meant I could not study biology in my final years at school, I would probably be a doctor now. I have been successful in many other fields - as a scientist, businesswoman, economist and musician, but I always promised myself that when my children were settled at school full-time I would fill the gap in my life sciences and apply to medical college. I am now studying biology and chemistry A-levels full time and I have never been happier. I have also had the good fortune to be able to shadow three GP's and one consultant, confirming my ambition to be an inner-city GP. I grew up surrounded by medicine (my grandmother was a GP and my grandfather a general surgeon) so I am very well aware of the commitment and deep sense of social responsibility that is needed in this profession.

The opening is weakened by beginning with an excuse. Emphasising the large number of roles they have had can be interpreted as lacking 'staying power' - a bit of a butterfly. In addition, the information is too densely packed - there is material for three paragraphs here.

Example 5:

Having been the sort of child who felt compelled, from an early age, to bandage her friends, rescue sick animals and avidly view TV hospital dramas, it was assumed by myself and my family that entering medicine was a foregone conclusion. However, the plans were somewhat disrupted by a sustained period of teenage rebellion, resulting in lower than expected O-level results. A-levels came to a sticky end at about the same time as my long-term boyfriend and two close family members. It was then I decided to take it easy with a medical secretarial course instead, and indulge in some essential paid employment, with the intention of resuming studies and attempting entrance to medical school when I felt better. During my second attempt at A-levels, I found myself unexpectedly pregnant, and decided I should do the decent thing and marry the father. Which, with hindsight, was a mistake because he was less than enthusiastic about my plans for world domination through medicine, and insisted that I settle for a quiet job as a secretary. I considered it a sensible option, as money was so scarce I could not afford to give up work and study anyway.

The use of a very informal style grabs the attention of the reader and their resilient, bubbly character shines through. However, the impact is marred by excuses.

Example 6:

I first became interested in a career in medicine when working in a boarding school. For two years I was responsible for Sick Wing during Matron's days off and during her sometimes protracted absences due to ill health. I routinely dealt with minor injuries and illnesses, liaising with the school GP or arranging for pupils to be taken to A&E if necessary. I was also responsible for administering non-prescription drugs and ensuring detailed accurate records were maintained.

Too old to be considered for medical school at that time, I was still interested in a career in science. I took two A levels in one academic year, relying on independent study because I was in a full time, resident post.

The opening paragraph is a straightforward description of relevant work experience and begins to answer 'why medicine?' even though this is some time in the past (as would be apparent from the work record - it is not necessary to highlight the timescale at this point on the form). The mention of extra A-levels and the circumstances under which they were taken in this case illustrates that the candidate has the motivation and discipline to study.

The Final Stages

Look again at the balance of your statement. How well have you used the space available to introduce yourself? Do you like this person? What is special about them? Keep checking actively for errors in spelling and grammar.

Once you are comfortable with your personal statement, make a printout formatted as for the UCAS form. Do not be tempted to squeeze in that last sentence by selecting a smaller font size than their stated minimum (12 point). The copy that the Admissions Tutor sees is tiny - your A3 form is reduced down to A4 - so avoid crowding the space allowed. Use mixed case if your statement is typed but select a clear font. 'Times' font is designed specifically for ease of reading.

If your personal statement is going to be handwritten, use a very fine black pen and print as clearly as you can in upper case throughout. Do not cover up errors with 'Tippex' or similar products - on the Admission Tutor's copy this will appear as a dense grey block and whatever is written over it is almost illegible.

Finally, check for adjacent lines beginning with the same word. The eye easily jumps a line under these circumstances and the reader may omit important information as a result. Restructure this part of your statement if necessary to avoid the problem.

Make one final printout. Do you like what you see? Are you happy for complete strangers to base their assumptions about you on this statement?

If so, complete the form and submit it on time.

Summary

DO NOT

    Make excuses

    Make errors in spelling and grammar

    Suggest that your current role is boring

    Repeat information found elsewhere on the form

    Overcrowd the space

    Dwell on the past

DO

    Make a strong opening statement

    Use clear, positive language throughout

    Focus on personal development

    Concentrate on the present

    Give a clear description of relevant work experience

Entrance Exams

The government drive for more doctors and wider access to medicine has resulted in new medical schools, new graduate entry courses and revised selection procedures. The increasingly large volume of applications, formulaic personal statements, high grades and lack of confidentiality with respect to references has made selecting candidates for interview increasingly difficult for all medical courses.

Amongst graduates, the age of applicants varies by over 20 years and many schools feel that the academic ability of such a variety of applicants cannot be measured by degree alone. The potential of a 21-year-old biochemistry graduate is incomparable with that of a 37-year-old lawyer. Entrance exams go some way towards levelling the playing field. For some people, the fact that their first class degree in biomedical sciences is almost irrelevant (for some schools) may be a source of frustration. However, schools hope to test skills and attitudes that are not directly measured in A-levels or undergraduate degree results.

Entry requirements for graduate entry programmes vary between schools far more than for standard course entry. Some schools feel that graduates of all disciplines should have the opportunity to apply, whilst others feel that a science background is essential. Study of the humanities has been shown to correlate with better clinical performance, but scientific knowledge is core to a medical degree. Of those schools requiring a science degree, some test science in their entrance exam, whilst others do not. Most schools accepting an arts degree test science in their entrance exam. However, King's College are notable in that they neither require a science degree, nor test science directly in their MSAT entrance exam. However, whilst the MSAT is not a science test as such, the responses given highlight whether the candidate has an aptitude for the logical reasoning and interpersonal skills required as a student and a clinician.

The format of each exam is broadly similar, with a predominance of multiple choice questions (MCQs). BMAT also uses extended matching questions (EMQs) and short answer questions (SAQs).

Please see Chapter 3 for entry requirements and statistics for each individual school.

Note that you must register for these exams in addition to the usual application to UCAS.

GAMSAT

The Graduate Australian Medical School Admissions Test (GAMSAT) has been developed by the Australian Council for Educational Research (ACER). The GAMSAT test, held in the UK on 6th January 2006 at a cost of £176, is being used by St George's University of London, University of Nottingham at Derby Medical School, Peninsula Medical School and the Clinical School at University of Wales, Swansea. It is the only tool that St George's and Nottingham use to assess academic performance for entry onto their graduate entry medical courses. Swansea uses GAMSAT as an additional tool to test academic performance for entry into its Graduate Entry Programme. Peninsula Medical School uses GAMSAT to assess the academic aptitude of prospective applicants who are not school leavers, for its 5-year MBBS programme. GAMSAT results are valid for 2 years. Candidates may sit the exam at centres in London, Birmingham, Bristol, Cardiff, Nottingham and Sheffield.

GAMSAT is divided into three sections, with a total test time of 5.5 hours designed to assess performance in the areas of:

1. *Reasoning in the Humanities and Social Sciences (75 MCQs in 100 minutes)*
2. *Written Communication (2 essays in 60 minutes)*
3. *Reasoning in Biological and Physical Sciences (110 MCQs in 170 minutes) (Chemistry 40%, Biology 40% and Physics 20%)*

Candidates must pass each section in addition to having an overall competitive score.

3 sets of GAMSAT sample papers and information booklet are available from UCAS www.ucas.co.uk

The information booklet can also be downloaded from www.acer.edu.au/tests/university/gamsatuk/intro.html

The deadline for application is 31st October 2005. The pdf version of the information booklet does not include a registration form, so you must obtain a hard copy from UCAS. Late registrations will be accepted up to 14th November 2005, on payment of a late fee of £47 in addition to the registration fee. You must fill in the form using a pencil, and must also submit one recent passport-sized photograph; the suggestion is a photograph that is less than six months old.

MSAT

The Medical School Admissions Test (MSAT) is held on 28th November 2005 at a cost of £75. The test is being used by King's College London, Queen Mary and Warwick University for their graduate entry fast track courses.

Like GAMSAT, ACER sets MSAT, but unlike GAMSAT, MSAT does not assess reasoning in basic sciences or the interpretation of complex verbal materials. It has a strong focus on general skills and personal attributes. It is designed to offer an alternative to GAMSAT for medical schools that do not wish to measure ability in the sciences directly, but instead wish to measure the general and personal skills and abilities which are less assessed in academic examinations. MSAT results are valid for 2 years. Candidates may sit the test at centres in London, Birmingham, Bristol, Cambridge and Sheffield.

MSAT consists of three discrete components, with a total test time of 3 hours designed to assess performance in the areas of:

> 1. *Critical Reasoning; general interest, basic science and social science (45 MCQs in 65 minutes)*
> 2. *Interpersonal Understanding (45 MCQs in 55 minutes)*
> 3. *Written Communication (2 essays in 60 minutes)*

The only ACER example questions available are found at www.acer.edu.au/tests/university/msat/intro.html

Unlike GAMSAT, registration is by online enrolment only. This opens mid- September and closes 28 October 2005, and should be completed at the website above. Late registrations will not be accepted. You will need an email address in order to register.

BMAT

The Biomedical Admissions Test (BMAT) is owned and administered by Cambridge Assessment, the new identity for University of Cambridge Local Examinations Syndicate. BMAT is held on 2nd November 2005, at a cost of £21.50, and is used by a number of schools for standard course entry. Only Cambridge uses this exam for selection for its graduate course. BMAT scores cannot be carried over to subsequent years.

BMAT consists of three discrete components, with a total test time of 2 hours designed to assess performance in the areas of:

    1. Aptitude and skills (35 MCQs and SAQs in 60 minutes)

    2. Scientific knowledge and application (27 MCQs and SAQs in 30 minutes)

    3. Written task (1 essay in 30 minutes)

The only Cambridge Assessment example questions available are found at the BMAT website www.bmat.org.uk This website also suggests reading materials.

The closing date for application is 30th September; late entries may be accepted between 1st - 15th October 2005 but will be charged late entry fees of £43.00 per candidate within the UK. There is a secure on-line entry system for registering for BMAT. If you are intending to take BMAT, you must register with an assessment centre, and not directly with BMAT. You can search for your nearest centre on the BMAT website.

Immediately after the BMAT exam, make a note of your essay subject and outline its content, as you may be required to discuss that essay at interview.

Oxford Entrance Exam

The admissions test for Oxford's graduate entry is different to the BMAT exam, and is administered by the Oxford Medical School. The test, held on 5th November in Oxford, is designed to provide a common standard against which an assessment can be made of candidates' skills in verbal and numerical comprehension and reasoning. It is only one of several indicators used to decide whether to shortlist candidates for interview. As such, Oxford test scores cannot be carried over to subsequent years. The exam consists of two discrete components, with a total test time of 2 hours designed to assess performance in the areas of:

1 a) Text comprehension (MCQs, SAQs and longer answers)

b) Possible essay (20 minute response to some text)

2. Numerical manipulation (SAQs)

The only Oxford example questions available are found at bmra.pharm.ox.ac.uk

The closing date for applications is 15th October 2005. Application forms are available from the Oxford Colleges Admissions Office. Late registrations will not be accepted.

General tips for MCQs and EMQs

Many teachers suggest reading the questions *prior* to the passage. This can be a very efficient use of time by allowing you to quickly filter through any redundant information.

- *Know before hand exactly how long you have for each question and stick to it.*
- *If you get stuck MOVE ON: you have about 1.5 min/question for GAMSAT science.*
- *Star any questions you feel you would like to revisit, but still answer them as it is unlikely that you will get back to them.*
- *Read the question(s) carefully: the information needed to answer is usually provided.*
- *The questions may occasionally be based on things that you are unlikely to have covered.*
- *If you are not familiar with something, try not to panic, but think about what principles they may be drawing on.*
- *You may want to jot down or highlight the key information given in the question.*
- *For some questions you may find it easier to exclude wrong answers than work out the correct answer.*
- *If you are unsure, make a reasoned guess as the papers are not negatively marked.*
- *Do not leave any questions unanswered. If necessary, spend the final 20 seconds of the exam simply blind guessing any remaining questions.*

- *Never leave an unfinished paper. Use the final 20 seconds to make utterly blind guesses for remaining questions if you have to.*

Exam Preparation

Often, suggestions of the required standard made by each examining board are rather vague, and the lack of any syllabus can leave candidates at a loss as to how to prepare. The exams are skills-based as much as knowledge-based. The aim of these exams is to test understanding and reasoning, not the candidate's ability to regurgitate lists of facts or equations. Of course, understanding is largely impossible without knowledge. Multiple choice questions (MCQs) in GAMSAT and MSAT, and further extended matching questions (EMQs) and short answer questions (SAQs) in BMAT and Oxford entrance, allow for a large number of unrelated questions and can therefore test a broad range of topics. A good way to revise for the graduate entrance exam papers is therefore to read as widely around a subject as possible, concentrating less on memorising hard facts and more on understanding basic principles and concepts. This approach should also help you to apply your knowledge, manipulate data and undertake critical reasoning.

However, knowledge will not only facilitate understanding, it will help you to answer the questions quickly, particularly in science sections. You should always know the amount of time available per question for any given paper and should practice answering questions within that time. Sample questions are available through UCAS, ACER and Cambridge Assessment and you should obtain these as soon as possible, to rate your starting ability, plan your revision and gain practice.

Suggested Reading

For the science sections, at least a strong A-level standard should be sought and ACER does recommend a first year degree level. Familiarity is more likely to result in understanding and skill than a last minute cram.

There is no safe answer to the question 'do I need to know this?' The genius may be able to quickly answer questions seemingly by a sixth sense, whilst another person may need extensive knowledge to answer what might seem to others to be common sense. The more reading you do, the better prepared you will be. Also, no knowledge is a waste, and any learning will be useful at medical school.

A study of the sample questions from the examining bodies should give you the best indication of where you should direct your efforts. However, the list below is based on the materials that have been used by a number of successful GAMSAT, MSAT, BMAT and Oxford entrance candidates. They are suggestions only; you will know best what type of material works for you, whether diagrammatic or text, internet or hard copy. The list below might help simply if you feel unable to find revision texts which are suitable for you.

Medical College Admission Test (MCAT) preparation guides

Although not specific to any UK entrance exam, many of the skills tested in the MCAT exam are very similar to those tested in ACER, Cambridge Assessment and Oxford medical school entrance exams. Note that MCAT candidates necessarily have a science degree and there is an emphasis on knowledge rather than just understanding. Note also that spelling and some terminology can be different in the US. However, these books cover natural sciences, maths, verbal reasoning and written communication.

Science Reading

Rather than rote learning scientific facts, aim to understand what you are reading. Make sure you have looked at sample questions from the GAMSAT and/or BMAT exam this should be the biggest factor in determining the extent of your study.

A-level revision guides:

Science Texts

1. *Oxford Revision Guides; AS+A-Level; www.oup.co.uk*
   - *very clear, with simple diagrams*
   - *the human biology book includes material used in first year graduate medicine*
   - *the physics book has a useful medical physics section*

2. *Revision Express; A-Level Study Guide (AS+A2); www.revision-express.com*
   - *slightly more wordy and more basic content than Oxford Revision Guides*
   - *excellent format of one topic per page*

3. *Letts Educational; A2 Level; www.letts-education.com*
   - *colourful and clear*
   - *great diagrams*
   - *excellent answer explanations*

4. *Make the Grade; AS+A2 Revision Guide; www.nelsonthornes.-com*
   - *simple style*

5. *Exam Revision Notes; AS/A-Level; www.philipallan.co.uk*
   - *very basic with minimal explanations*
   - *revision notes only*

Basic Science Internet guides.

There are lots of internet-based revision and learning sites, many of which are listed on: www.dulwich.org.uk/gateway/revision.html

Many sites are rather gimmicky, but they are a great resource for people feeling a little overwhelmed and frightened by the whole science issue.

Also, they can be great for dipping into for just 10 minutes a day at work.

Skills in Reasoning
Reasoning skills depend on using logic i.e. drawing conclusions on the basis of evidence before you.

Critical reasoning (MSAT)
You will need to apply problem solving skills in this component. Usually, the kind of skills you draw on will be almost intuitive but if you are stuck, use rough paper to work out what is required, then assess whether your answer can be supported by the evidence before you.

Interpersonal skills (MSAT)
You will be presented with some dialogue and asked to comment on the use of language by one of the parties in the dialogue. You will not have non-verbal communication to help you so it is important to 'listen' to what is being said. Try reading it to yourself as if you were reading aloud.

Reasoning in the humanities and social sciences (GAMSAT)
You will face a number of questions with multiple choice answers. If you read the questions before you read the passages, you will focus better on the passage with a view to seeking the correct answer. Again, you will be presented with data in different formats and your task is to interpret this data correctly.

Comprehension in BMAT
BMAT seems keen on syllogisms and varieties of syllogisms so make sure you understand the traps in this form of argument e.g.

True/False question:
The sun rose today

The sun rose yesterday
Therefore the sun will rise tomorrow.

Further Reading for Reasoning
The links below may offer you some suggestions for improving your reasoning:

> *commhum.mccneb.edu/argument/summary.htm*
> *To do: read and work through exercises*

> *www.fallacyfiles.org/*
> *To do: read the section on 'What is a fallacy', 'Fallacy Watch' and 'Fallacy Examples'*

> *www.datanation.com/fallacies/*
> *To do: read 'Index of the Logical Fallacies'*

Skills in Written Communication
The purpose of the essay is to see whether you can assemble a set of ideas in a coherent manner in a short space of time.

Whatever the type of essay, there are three parts to a successful essay: planning, paragraphing and sticking to the point. Remember, you only have 30 minutes for the essay.

Planning
- *Take up to 10 minutes in the planning.*
- *Read the brief carefully and think of three points to make. Write these down.*
- *Under each point, make some notes to explain and expand the point.*

Paragraphing

- *You need about five or so paragraphs: introduction, the three points above and a conclusion.*
- *Usually each paragraph contains a single idea.*
- *The conclusion is drawn from the main point of each paragraph.*

Stick to the point
- *Keep to your plan.*
- *Check that you have covered the points you wished to make.*
- *Check that your conclusion is drawn from the points in each paragraph.*

Written Communication for GAMSAT

There are two types of essay in this test: reflective (personal) and objective (less personal). Read the following and decide which essay type you are more comfortable with.

The reflective essay asks you to reveal your own feelings. You can do this as a response to a topic and ensure you give examples e.g. in a topic such as 'travel broadens the mind', you should give examples of how travel changed your views so you need to state what the views were and how they were changed through the experience of travel.

The more objective essay will ask you to explore a view on something. Again, produce a few points, exemplify them and come to a conclusion (which might be that there is no conclusion!)

Written Communication for MSAT

There are two parts to this question: a response to some quotations, and text supporting some data.

Quotation

Usually three quotes will be given and you are expected to write a response. You can use all three quotes (often they will be contradictory) or you can write a response to one. The purpose of this exercise is to find out what you make of the quotes. The same rules as above apply: make some notes, put these into paragraphs, write an introduction and a conclusion.

Interpretation of data

This task is to assess your understanding of data presented in graphical form. Essentially you are asked to write a commentary on the data presented.

You will be given some data such as statistics and/or a graph or tables. Your task is to assess and analyse the data and draft a commentary. Sometimes the data will not be comparative (e.g. uses different datasets) so you need to be able to say that valid comparisons cannot be made. This task does not require specialist knowledge of statistics so avoid using specialist statistical terms.

Written Communication for BMAT

The written communication component of BMAT is very specific so you must read the brief very carefully and follow it to the letter. To a large extent, the paragraph headings are to be found in the brief, so you must answer and amplify the questions posed but beware of giving a mechanical answer; it is your response that the examiners are anxious to read.

Further Reading for Written Communication

The links below may offer you some suggestions for improving your essay writing technique.

www.bbc.co.uk/learning/returning/betterlearner/studyskills/j_essays_01.shtml
To do: read and make notes on the points relevant to your own essay writing

You will find further ideas about essay writing on some of the forums, e.g. the 'essay writing for GAMSAT' section at www.medschoolguide.co.uk Note that the postings are subjective opinions and may not always be accurate - you must use a critical eye.

There are numerous study guides which include sections on essay writing. One book with a simple clear approach is found in Derek Rowntree, *Learn How to Study: a realistic approach* 4th edition (Warner, 1998)

See also Flesch, Rudolph; Lass, A.H., *A Classic Guide to Better Writing* (New York: Harper, 1966) and make sure you have the latest edition.

Commercial Preparation Courses
Although the entrance examinations afford broader opportunities to many graduates, an individual's background can have a bearing on their ability. Some candidates have been successful in the GAMSAT exam on second and even third attempts, simply through perseverance and greater preparation. In addition to private study, taught options open to candidates include night school and preparation courses with private companies. It is a reasonable argument made by some schools that graduates seeking a place on a highly self-directed graduate medicine course should be more than capable of self-directing their study for the purposes of the entrance exams. Conversely, graduates should be mature adults who are capable of choosing which resources work well for them and that good teaching and extra practice can greatly support private study. Additional 'mock' papers are available from a number of companies found on the internet. Remember that there is no association between private companies and the schools or examining boards. Therefore, schools are not in a position to either endorse or criticise any commercial options. Similarly, there can be no guarantee from any company as to how closely their mock exam papers will match the real thing, nor should they be privy to any confidential information.

However, many students on graduate medical courses today have found commercial products and services to be invaluable.

Useful items to take to the exams.
- *Passport or photo driving licence originals, not photocopies*
- *Admission ticket*
- *Map of how to get there. Allow time for possible public transport problems, whether technical, environmental or security.*
- *Do not make firm arrangements for the evening GAMSAT over-ran by 2 hours one year*
- *Limit your valuables security has been variable*
- *Ear plugs*
- *Calculator but not for BMAT and Oxford Entrance*
- *Umbrella people have had to queue in the rain in the past*
- *Additional jumper it is hard to control the temperature in an enormous hall*
- *Tissues*
- *Pens, pencil, ruler - to underline your essay titles*
- *Sugary sweets*
- *Water*

The Interview

Although the interview is a stand-alone final hurdle, it is the culmination of all your efforts so far. As such, we will discuss here not only final preparation and practice, but also the concepts, attitudes and experiences you should have dwelt on in the months, if not years, preceding the interview.

You will often hear, not least from the medical schools, that preparing for interview can be a risky activity. Preparation is a broad term which covers everything from work experience to practising answers, to familiarising oneself with the format. The concern of admissions tutors does not relate so much to preparation as to 'coaching'. Preparation and practice is undertaken by successful candidates, whilst coaching can be counterproductive. Coaching implies that candidates are primed with 'correct' answers. There is hardly ever a single correct answer, regurgitation is rarely endearing, and such candidates may not have the skills to answer a question for which they were not coached.

We encourage preparation and practice and will not provide you with any supposed 'correct' answers.

What are the schools looking for?
Graduate candidates, particularly, should be focused on the fact that they are applying for a career, not just a degree. This attitude is appropriate, after all the interviewers are looking for potential doctors rather than just medical students.

The numerous qualities that are sought in potential doctors are highlighted in *Tomorrow's Doctors* and in the medical school prospectuses. Throughout this book, and particularly in chapters 2, 6 and 7, many qualities are discussed which you might hope to demonstrate at interview. You may find it useful to revisit those chapters now.

To name but a few, these qualities include:

Genuine interest in Medicine
- *Commitment to medicine*
- *Motivation towards a medical career*
- *Realistic view of the role of a doctor*
- *Appreciation of the medical school's course design*

Personal attributes
- *Communication (written, listening and speaking)*
- *Communication with people of different backgrounds*
- *Communication of difficult information*
- *Broad social, cultural or sporting interests*
- *A well-rounded personality*
- *Empathy, compassion and patience*
- *Caring attitude and concern for the welfare of others*
- *Non judgemental*
- *Interest in People*
- *A respect for people and their rights, dignity and opinions*
- *Integrity*
- *What you can offer the medical school*
- *Ability to self-criticise and know one's strengths and weakness*
- *Humility and an open mind*

Skills

- *Academic knowledge*
- *Willingness to keep updated*
- *Ability to describe and discuss important issues in medicine*
- *Capacity for self-directed knowledge acquisition*
- *Willingness to accept responsibility*
- *Practical Skills*
- *Ability to learn and implement new ideas and skills*
- *Organisational skills*
- *Non-academic accomplishments*
- *Problem-solving skills*

Team player

- *Realisation of other health professionals' roles*
- *Teamwork*
- *Leadership*

Coping under stress

- *Recognition of the stresses in medicine*
- *Recognition of stress in oneself and others*
- *Ability to recognise limitations*
- *Strategies for coping*

You might now be eager to know how to demonstrate the above qualities at interview, but the practicalities of how you will do this will in part vary on the structure of your interview.

Types of Interview Structure

Structured - notably Nottingham and St George's
These interviews are extremely structured: all candidates are asked the same questions. Therefore, your interviewers almost certainly will not

ask questions that follow naturally from your first response (although they will ask open questions that allow *you* to pick examples from your repertoire). This can feel extremely unnerving and you might wonder if they have listened to a word. You may also find that your smile is not reciprocated. The reason for strictly-structured interviews is simply that it is a fair process and allows a more objective scoring system. All candidates are asked the same open questions and no conversation ensues.

For instance, a question testing your ability to communicate might be: 'Tell us about a time when you have had to communicate difficult information.' The interviewers are looking for more than just an example. Without prompt, you need to offer your analysis of that example, what you did well or poorly and what you learned from it. Since your answers cannot be debated, you should strive to offer other points of view. This approach might sound like an abuse of your air time, and will be in striking contrast to a normal two-way conversation but, of course, if you consider that follow-up questions will not be asked, you need to give all the information first time around. At most, they will ask 'Anything else?' Remember that this does not mean that there *should* be something else; it is simply their way of checking that you are ready to move on.

St George's and Nottingham run their selection procedure jointly. Candidates are called to interview based on their GAMSAT score. Candidates who apply to both schools will be interviewed once and could receive no, one or two offers.

Semi-structured

Most interviews are semi-structured. The bulk of questions will be prepared in advance, as with a structured interview. However, the interview is likely to develop into a more normal conversation, which could include reference to your personal statement. The conversational environment can feel less daunting, but does mean that your answers can be debated so be very careful not to contradict yourself or your personal statement. The big advantage can be that you can leave signposts at the end of your response such that *you* guide the interview. Nice trick, but do not rely on it - the interviewers may ignore your attempt to lead the interview. Also, do not be lazy in the light of conversation - you can still pre-empt the ensuing questions. Answer as fully as is advised for a structured interview, by giving evidence to support your answer, or by volunteering another way of thinking about things, for example.

Unstructured

In a completely unstructured interview, the questions are relatively, or totally, unprepared. They may include similar questions to those often found in structured interviews, or questions developed from your personal statement, or they may follow a completely tortuous and random route. Bear in mind that all the interviewers are likely to be looking for the same skills and attributes, so prepare as much as you can, and consider the arguments to your responses.

Stations

Queen Mary use a series of stations. Candidates spend 10 minutes in each station, where each station deals with a different skill that the school is looking for. You might also be played a video and/or given material to read in advance of a station, which will then be discussed.

Availability of your UCAS form to the interviewers

This generally coincides with how structured the interview is. If the interviewers are asking everyone the same question (structured), it is impossible to ask something that relates to your personal statement or exam results. For some interviews, the interviewers are blinded to your personal statement and UCAS information. This means that the interviewer knows absolutely nothing about you. You must work into your interview anything that you feel they should know, irrespective of how eloquently you described it in your personal statement. Even for those schools that will read your personal statement, you should bear in mind that it is unlikely to be read in detail. You would be well-advised to divulge at interview that valuable information found within your personal statement, and expand on it.

Schools whose interviewers will have seen your UCAS personal statement (or other supplementary forms) prior to interview

Birmingham	*Yes*
Bristol	*Yes*
Cambridge	*Yes*
King's	*No*
Leicester	*Yes*
Liverpool	*Yes*
Newcastle	*Yes*
Nottingham	*No*
Oxford	*Yes*
Queen Mary	*Yes*
Southampton	*n/a*
St George's	*No*
Swansea	*Yes*
Warwick	*Unknown*

N.B. King's will use your personal statement for consideration for the standard entry course.

Organising your tool box before interview
If you have ever filled in one of the long 'milk round' style application forms for private sector jobs, you will be familiar with a series of six or so questions in the style of 'give us an example of a time when you have ...'

such as worked under stress, accepted responsibility, worked in a team, communicated difficult information and so on. You may have an equivalent number of experiences that you would like to tell them about as questions. Whilst your best experience is often applicable to more than one of the questions, you have to arrange the examples to produce the optimal combination. It is not so easy with an interview, since you want to include your prize experience, whilst at the same time not using it too soon such that you cannot answer a subsequent question. You might find it useful to create a table, with necessary qualities as the rows, and your experiences as columns, and try to assign one experience to each quality or skill. You may find that tidying up your virtual toolbox will help you to recall useful experiences in the pressure of the moment.

Although all medical schools are essentially looking for the same skills, the emphasis placed on each one can be different for each school. Make sure that you read the school prospectus carefully to gauge the weighting and confirm the interview's structure, length, and number of interviewers.

Practice discussing each of the required skills out loud and to anyone that will listen. Discuss why the skills are important. Do you have these skills? What is your evidence?

How to answer a question!
There are some key themes which you can consider employing to assist you in putting forward a well structured response. A good argument is one which is both sound (that the steps follow logically) and valid (that you are accurate). To put this into practice, we will consider three aspects of your response. Firstly, your form - here we mean the nature and quality of your speech as well as body language. Secondly, your structure - flow and categorisation. Thirdly, your content - the importance of comments that are accurate, relevant and supported with evidence.

Form

This is the hardest of the three aspects for you to analyse and even harder to correct. It is also fundamentally important. If you are inaudible, or sit scratching your privates, you will struggle to compete.

The key here is to practice and get feedback. Everyone's opinion of your performance is valid - are you making sense? Does your practice interviewer visualise someone like you advising them on their medical care? For the first time, pay attention to your mother - if she has always scolded you for running your hands through your hair, now is the time to consider that she might be right. Similarly, do not only seek advice from those people you are sure will give you only positive feedback, seek criticism too. The best person to approach is probably the one you are most embarrassed to ask! Ask a medical person to give you a practice interview. Some people choose to go on interview practice courses.

Structure

Structure is most important in a structured interview, but the skills discussed here are useful to consider in any good communication.

How often have you thought, or said, 'that came out wrong?' Or confused a friend because you had changed subject without indicating that change? Or had to back track, saying 'sorry, I should have explained that bit first?' This is an easy area to make big improvements. Think before you start! Pause for longer than feels natural - the gaping pause you feel will not seem as long to the interviewers, who will respect you for thinking about their well-thought-out question. Feel free to say 'I will just think about that for a moment.' Even if you are not surprised by the question, still pause. It might be subtly different from your immediate assumption.

Many people find it helpful to categorise what they are about to say. 'There are 3 aspects to my answer X,Y,Z. In terms of X,...' Chunking in this way makes your reply easier to follow, and gives you, and the interviewers, a framework in advance. Alternatively, follow the same rules as you were taught for essay writing at school. Give an introduction, evidence (categorisation could equally come in here) and conclusion.

Whenever you give broad headings or a list, by way of an introduction, you should then give examples, particularly in a structured interview. Anyone can give a list, but what does communication, say, mean to you? Describe the doctor who really listened to your concerns about your spots when you were a teenager. Tell of the time when you witnessed sad news being broken well (or badly) to a relative. Tell of the skills you identified in a doctor you shadowed who was particularly good at communication. This book cannot give you your examples, it can merely suggest that you have them and use them.

Content
Answer the question! Do not be a politician and answer what you would have liked them to have asked. This may sound obvious, but it is extremely tempting to give your perfectly-prepared answer to a surprise question that you have never thought of. Pausing before answering will reduce the risk of this occurring.

You can answer the surprisingly nasty question well though - pause, think, chunk your response, be yourself, be honest, and then stop. Do not verbally wander the recesses of your mind for something profound, just answer the question and move on.

Do not feel under pressure to provide astounding experiences. Indeed, you may be able to better demonstrate your personal attributes if you describe what it means to you to help an old lady cross the road than dramatising the time when you saved a celebrity from choking with much applause from nearby diners.

Also, try to keep a balance. Being so overwhelmed with empathy towards death and suffering that you never express any joy can really depress your interviewers. They will not want to work with someone who depresses them for the entire interview remember the really great things too.

Common Mistakes & things to bear in mind

Speaking too fast

Slowing down will not only help to avoid exhausting your interviewers, you will probably deliver your information more concisely and will automatically improve your structure and content.

Being defensive

Classics examples of this for graduate entry courses are thinking that you are too old and instead of answering ıwhy do you want to study medicine?ı the question the older candidate obviously heard was ıwhy do you think you have got enough marbles left to do this, you old fool?ı The decision to interview you means that your age does not preclude you from studying, and that means that lots of very wise, experienced (and old) people have sat around a big table deciding that old folks like you can be just as valuable as the young ones. Of course, older candidates need to show a greater degree of commitment, but that comes from passion, enthusiasm and experience, not a defensive attitude and a biography of your failures.

Similarly, if you are specifically asked at interview why your A-level results are so horribly bad, again, resist the temptation to offer excuses. You might offer something along the lines of, ıWell, there were family/ personal problems for me at the time but ultimately I did not work hard enough and got the results I deserved.ı By accepting responsibility, you will have demonstrated maturity, honesty and an ability to develop yourself.

Nervous habits

You cannot necessarily stop yourself from going bright red, but you can avoid nail biting, neck scratching, mouth covering, hand wringing, ceiling gazing and nervous laughing.

Not smiling

A fixed smile is horrid, of course, but if you are answering a question in which you are describing your enthusiasm for medicine, a cold, blank face does not help to convince the examiners of that enthusiasm.

Being Arrogant

You do not know everything there is to know about anything.

Being patronising / too technical

Demonstrate your communication skills by pitching your answers appropriately. You should be introduced at the start of the interview. Try to remember each interviewer's profession; you may even be able to involve them in your answer more: 'I imagine you see that sort of thing in your department all the time.'

Interviewers get very nervous too!

The really blank faced nasty one could later be a great colleague and friend.

Being really stuck

You may *really* draw a complete blank on a question, for instance: ιtell us about a time when you have had to take on responsibility. Answer as far as you can, indicating to the interviewers how you have changed the question. You might approach it by saying, 'I'm sure I have an example to give you but my mind has gone blank; however, thinking about how other people handle responsibility' You may be able to show insight into how a colleague handled responsibility well and why that skill is important in a doctor. If that does not get you rolling, just explain what you think responsibility means. Make it snappy, indicating your need to move on: 'that's as much as I can think of right now', and let it go.

It is true that they are not there to catch you out
Equally, do not set yourself up for a fall by (for instance) being arrogant, saying you are interested in something you know nothing about, or saying that you do not like what you are doing at the moment because you do not like needy people.

Do not be fazed by people making notes/scores
It is a fair process for you. And for goodness sake do not try to look at them! You are trying to embark on a career with necessarily high standards of professional conduct - you do not want to look like a cheat. Look at your interviewer instead. Also, seeing the scores will not help you - is the highest score 1 or 10?

Try to get a balance between being over and under prepared
There is an easy solution to being under prepared of course - prepare. If you are over prepared, try to relax, try to feel the emotions that you are describing. You do not want to be describing what a death in your family meant to you with a voice normally saved for shopping list recital.

Try not to be a walking dictionary
Long lists of abbreviations/names of departments/consultants are not impressive. Also, there may be non-medical people on the panel. Remain human and endearing.

Example Questions
The questions here have been picked not so much for their frequency of occurrence, but in order to demonstrate common skills applied in such answers.

What makes a good doctor?

The qualities described at the start of this chapter should provide some ideas upon which to build your answer. However, do not simply recite a list - anyone can do that. Your answer should be framed in the light of your work experience and you should have developed your own understanding. If you develop examples from your experiences, you will demonstrate commitment and insight.

Why do you want to change to medicine at this stage?

This question is not *"why have you failed before?"*, or *"aren't you too old?"* There is no reason to be defensive. Have respect and appreciation for your current profession, explain how medicine provides additional benefits to you now, view your maturity positively, be realistic but not negative and simply describe your motivation. You should have a positive answer to any question which asks why you *want* to do something.

Tell us about a particularly stressful time in your life, work or personal, and how you coped with it.

Again, your interviewers are looking for more than just an example. They are looking for insight, and a demonstration of skills. Explain why the experience is relevant to medicine. Remember that everyone found their first degree stressful; most graduates have something better that they can discuss.

What work and voluntary experience have you had which would help you to become a good doctor and help you in your studies?

Again, do not bore your interviewers with a list. Similarly, do not be showy about whom you have worked with. Also, do not act as though you know everything there is to know about the area of medicine that you witnessed. Being arrogant is not a useful attribute in a doctor. Be humble and enthusiastic, 'paint pictures' of memorable patients and interesting things that you have witnessed, or skills that you were able to demonstrate.

What pressures do you think doctors face in their professional and personal lives?
Again, this question should be framed in the light of your work experience and you should have developed your own understanding and insight. Pressures that you may have witnessed, and can expand on, might include: hard work (as a student or doctor), hours worked, uncooperative/ungrateful patients, difficult colleagues, death and suffering, management and political pressures (e.g. rationing), safety, relationship pressures, an increasingly litigious society, etc.

Explain a time when you have had to communicate difficult information.
With this type of question, do try to pick a good example. We have actually heard one candidate describe how difficult it was to communicate some rather sensitive information *in a text message*. Demonstrate that you recognise what is good communication and why it is important for a doctor to communicate well. Be humble and acknowledge what you learnt from the experience and what you could have done differently.

Current Affairs and Advances in Medicine
You may be asked if there is anything of a medical nature that has interested you in the news lately. It is not useful for us to attempt to summarise current affairs here. You should have a broad understanding of many topics in health, science, finance, politics and ethics relating to healthcare, and a more detailed understanding of a few issues. Websites at the end of this chapter will be a great source of further reading, in addition to an overview of information in the newspapers - which is of course what patients read. Try to think about the different aspects of what you read - what does your topic mean to patients, relatives, doctors, NHS finances, public health, ethics and so on.

Ethical Dilemmas

Some schools (e.g. Cambridge and King's) use an ethical case study, or clinical scenario to test your attitude towards working in the NHS. They will look for realism and a balanced outlook. You will probably be given time to look at your scenario. You will probably have a gut reaction and a sense of what is right, but try to see different points of view and potential flaws in your argument. Whilst offering your opinion will inform the interviewers of your outlook, an empathy for different views is useful, not least because your opinion could be deemed wrong.

You may be pushed until your knowledge and ideas are exhausted. This does not mean that the interviewers do not like you. Indeed, it could mean that they are enjoying the discussion with you. Equally, do not become argumentative when pushed. As a doctor, you would have to remain calm and professional, to listen to the views of others, and be willing to accommodate those views.

Consider the following scenario:

A 15 year old girl undergoes an emergency operation for the removal of an ectopic pregnancy (a dangerous pregnancy outside the womb). She asks you not to tell her mother anything. The mother demands to know what has happened to her daughter.

You may or may not know the current requirements relating to confidentiality, and it does not matter - the interviewer is likely to be most interested in how laterally you are able to think and how well you are able to structure and present your response.

The notes below are not prescriptive or exhaustive, but simply ideas that one might consider developing in an answer.

- *Identify that this is a dilemma about confidentiality*
- *Identify that the girl is a patient*
- *Identify that the patient is a minor*
- *Identify that the pregnancy is the result of statutory rape*
- *To what extent is this abuse who is the father?*
- *Consider when it might be appropriate to disclose patient information*
- *Should the mother be informed?*
- *Should the police be informed?*
- *This will lead you to your dilemma*

  a) a patient is owed a duty of confidentiality it is the very essence of the patient/doctor relationship

  b) is a mother allowed information regarding her daughter's medical care when that daughter is below a certain age?

- *If you know about confidentiality, competence, consent and disclosure you can offer more evidence about what should be considered do not worry if you do not know about these things, you will learn about them at medical school!*
- *It is likely that you will not know the precise answer to your dilemma; otherwise it would not be a very good dilemma! So, debate the issue and offer your own personal opinion in a non-judgemental way.*
- *It can be a nice conclusion to say that whilst you have offered your personal opinion, that you understand that you will be working within guidelines that may not always meet with your own personal opinion.*

(For more information, see www.gmc-uk.org/standards and follow the links to guidance and confidentiality and in particular sections 36-39. You might also follow the links to consent and children (section 23). This is an excellent site to gain a broad understanding of many ethico-legal issues.)

Asking Questions of the Interviewer

An interviewer will often conclude the interview by inviting you to ask any questions. This is not an indication that you *ought* to, or that they feel you *should* say something now that you did not say earlier. They are courteously providing you with an opportunity to ask a specific question, should you have one, and nothing else. Do not see it as an opportunity to give yourself more time and another opportunity to engage the interviewers in new detail. If you ask a question, do not ask for information that is available in the prospectuses or should have been obtained prior to application. They will have another interview to do after you, and would probably rather get on with it, so avoid unnecessary questions. Whether you ask a question or not, always thank the interviewer(s) for their time.

On the day
- *Arrive on time*
- *Make sure that you have read the prospectus and know about the course and the medical school.*
- *Wear smart clothes, tie your hair back, note your posture (especially in a skirt), and take care with body odour.*
- *In the interview, you must be honest, sincere, confident, relaxed, and positive. You need to inspire confidence in your ability to succeed in medical school and to become a compassionate and skilled physician. It is important to communicate why you be-lieve you are a qualified candidate and what you have done to prepare for medical school.*

Further help

- *www.bma.org,*
- *www.thelancet.com*
- *www.gmc-uk.org*
- *www.bmj.com*
- *www.studentbmj.com*
- *www.who.int*
- *www.direct.gov.uk*
- *www.nejm.org*

And Finally

We hope that this book will help you to secure a place at medical school. We wish you the best of luck in your studies and look forward to meeting a few of you during your training. However, the sad fact is that most applicants will not secure a place. Whilst it would not be appropriate for some candidates in particular to be awarded a place at medical school, many unsuccessful applicants have great potential and may well succeed on subsequent attempts. Some of the best graduate entry medical students that we have encountered admitted to having applied in three consecutive years before receiving an offer.

Age not withstanding, you might consider treating your unsuccessful applications as a learning opportunity. You will have undertaken some, if not all, of the following: work experience, the completion of application forms, preparation for and completion of entrance exams and interviews. This experience is enormously valuable try - to remember how daunted and uninformed you were when you started this process.

Above all, learn from your mistakes. Could you have started work experience sooner? Could you have found more valuable work experience? Did you get the most out of that work experience? Were you able to think deeply about patients, the pros and cons of medicine, and about yourself? Did you prepare adequately for the exams? Did you practise all the sample papers? Did you practise writing timed essays? Did anyone feed back to you on the standard of those essays? Did you frequently verbalise your medical aspirations and gain feedback on whether your desire and insight was apparent?

Few candidates prepare as well as they could, including the successful ones. If you have been through the process once, you have an advantage over the candidate who is navigating their way for the first time. Of course, we hope that this book goes a long way to ensuring that candidates do not feel lost in their application year, or indeed as they embark upon their training and beyond.

There are options for studying medicine other than graduate entry, of course. You may consider a standard entry course, an overseas course, a foundation programme or an access to medicine course. These options are distinct from graduate entry and will therefore not be discussed here. However, if you feel that you have exhausted your efforts in applying to graduate entry courses, you may find that there are other options available to you.

We wish you all the best in the pursuit of your vocation.